Praise for Beyond Lyme Disease

Connie Strasheim is a leading author i... ...th-er chronic health issues. Her latest bou... ...se: **Heal-ing the Underlying Causes of Chronic I... ... with Borreliosis and Co-Infections**, presents much neede... ...ination; bridging the gap between chronic Lyme disease and a myriad of other health conditions that may concurrently be causing "dis-ease" in an individual.

While it is easy to think of Lyme disease infections as being the sole cause of illness, Connie's groundbreaking book paints a much more comprehensive and realistic picture – that there are numerous factors at work; numerous pieces of a very complex puzzle. From adrenal fatigue to mold toxins, electromagnetic radiation and nutrient deficiencies, Connie evaluates the role that such imbalances can play in one's health. Evaluating and addressing these other factors may be key in recovery from chronic illness and may be grossly under-recognized to date.

Connie's view that Lyme disease may be just one piece of a larger puzzle is insightful and highly relevant, clinically. No one factor is the sole cause of disease; many factors are at play. Connie has combined her extensive medical knowledge with her own personal experiences to produce a much-needed work that will help many people who suffer from Lyme disease and other chronic illness.

—Nicola Mc Fadzean, N.D., Naturopathic Physician

Beyond Lyme Disease not only serves as a roadmap for the patient with Lyme disease, but could also be a standalone book on integrative medicine. Connie Strasheim's knowledge of the subject is quite extensive, both as an author and fellow survivor of Lyme disease. She covers many topics, ranging from nutrition, to GI and adrenal dysfunction; heavy metal toxicity, parasites, mold toxicity and electromagnetic radiation. She explores those topics that are of concern to all of us, and explains how they can affect patients who have the added burden of Lyme disease and its associated illnesses. She also helps patients to look at the factors that can undermine their health and healing.

Connie gives the reader a great foundation from which to start an integrative treatment protocol for their condition. This foundation can enable patients to look at how they are doing presently; the treatments that they might want to consider doing for their health, and how they can work with a Lyme-literate or integrative health care practitioner to start implementing those changes to their health.

I believe that patients who have access to this book will be so much better informed and will better understand the rationale behind their different treatment options, which will in turn facilitate the job of healing for both them and their doctors.

—Steven Bock, MD

Beyond
Lyme
Disease

BioMed Publishing Group

P.O. Box 550531

South Lake Tahoe, CA 96155

www.LymeBook.com

Copyright 2012 by Connie Strasheim

For related books and DVDs, visit us online at www.LymeBook.com.

ISBN: 978-0-9825138-9-7

DISCLAIMER

This book is not intended as medical advice. It is also not intended to prevent, diagnose, treat or cure disease. Instead, the book is intended only to share the unofficial research and opinion of the author. The book is provided for informational and educational purposes only, not as treatment instructions for any disease. Much of the book is a statement of opinion in areas where the facts are controversial or do not exist. The information in this book should not be considered any more valid than any other type of informal opinion.

The book was not written to replace the advice or care of a qualified health care professional. Be sure to check with your own qualified health care provider before beginning any protocols or procedures discussed in this book, or before stopping or altering any diet, lifestyle, or other therapies previously recommended to you by your health care provider. The treatments described in this book may have side effects and carry other known and unknown risks and health hazards.

Lyme disease is a controversial topic and this book should not be seen as the final word regarding Lyme disease medical care. The statements in this book have not been evaluated by the United States FDA.

Beyond
Lyme
Disease

Healing the Underlying Causes of Chronic Illness in People with Borreliosis and Co-Infections

Connie Strasheim

Foreword by

Lee Cowden, MD

Also by Connie Strasheim

Insights Into Lyme Disease Treatment: 13 Lyme-Literate Health Care Practitioners Share Their Healing Strategies

Defeat Cancer: 15 Doctors of Integrative & Naturopathic Medicine Tell You How

The Lyme Disease Survival Guide: Physical, Lifestyle, and Emotional Strategies for Healing

Healing Chronic Illness: By His Spirit, Through His Resources

Available to purchase from:

www.LymeBytes.Blogspot.com

■|) *Contents*

FOREWORD vii

PREFACE xiii

CHAPTER 1   Adrenal Insufficiency and
            Hypothyroidism..................................1

CHAPTER 2   Nutrient Deficiencies and Toxic Food...........23

CHAPTER 3   Electromagnetic Radiation/Pollution............53

CHAPTER 4   Mold and Mycotoxins.................................75

CHAPTER 5   Pyroluria/Heavy Metal Toxicity.....................93

CHAPTER 6   Parasites...111

CHAPTER 7   Gastrointestinal Dysfunction.......................123

CHAPTER 8   Emotional Trauma and Depression..............133

CHAPTER 9   Other Conditions That Contribute to Disease
            in People with Tick-Borne Infections............ 159

➤ Candida (and other types of fungal overgrowth).. 160

➤ Opportunistic viruses, bacteria, and other
  pathogens...164

➤ Foci infections in the mouth............................167

➤ Other environmental toxins and compromised
  detoxification mechanisms................................172

➤ Structural problems..177

APPENDIX I   Information and Tips on Diagnosing and
             Treating Tick-Borne Infections.....................187

APPENDIX II Babesia and Bartonella Symptoms
             and Indicators.. 207

Foreword to Beyond Lyme Disease
—*Lee Cowden, MD*

In my experience as a physician treating Lyme patients, I have discovered that when Lyme is affecting a patient, other conditions are also affecting their health. Hence, if all we ever do is "kill bugs," the patient may never get well. In Beyond Lyme Disease, Connie has started a very important discussion – not about Lyme co-infections, but about Lyme co-conditions. She has also done a great job explaining why so many people with Borreliosis and co-infections remain ill and symptomatic, even after what should be sufficient treatment for these infections. She has taken on a difficult subject and made it quite understandable.

As you read this book, I would encourage you to take note of the other factors that can contribute to Lyme disease. She points out, in an easy-to-understand way, how various co-existing conditions can keep people ill, often with symptoms that mimic Lyme disease. These conditions may have even preceded the development of Lyme and/or predisposed such people to the onset of Lyme disease, and include: adrenal and thyroid insufficiency, mold and/or mycotoxin exposure, nutrient deficiencies, toxic and/or allergenic foods, electromagnetic pollution, pyroluria, heavy metal toxicity, parasitism, gastrointestinal dysfunction, emotional trauma, candidiasis, opportunistic viruses and bacteria, oral foci infections, structural misalignments, and environmental toxins. These factors have the potential by themselves to make a person severely ill and some can even cause death. To focus solely on "bugs" to the exclusion of these other factors is foolhardy.

Beyond Lyme Disease has good references to support its assertions, plus other extremely useful information on the diagnosis and treatment of Borreliosis and co-infections in the Appendix. I believe that not only patients who are struggling with Lyme disease symptoms will benefit from the information in this book, but also the health professionals who are trying to help them. It is my hope that patients and practitioners alike will take the issues presented in this book to heart so that more and more people will be able to overcome their illnesses.

"How do I get over Lyme?" is a common question among those who have Lyme disease, but in reality, there is a much more appropriate question that they should be asking, which is, "How do I get well?" *Beyond Lyme Disease* has answers to that very important question. And Connie has done a great job in providing readers with the missing tools that they need to get well.

I have known Connie for several years as an author, speaker, advocate, and most importantly, as a spiritual sister and friend. In order to trust the content of any published work, you must be able to trust the author. I trust Connie and I agree with the concepts she has conveyed in this book.

Lyme disease is not well-understood in the medical community. It not only imitates other diseases, but can also be very difficult to diagnose. In the search to discover the source of their discomfort and pain, many people feel such a sense of relief when they are finally given a Lyme diagnosis, that they quit exploring why they feel as badly as they do, even though they are being affected by other significant conditions and symptoms not directly associated with Lyme.

In general, society doesn't understand Lyme, either, and many people with the disease do not receive the same empathy and compassion that people with other diseases such as breast cancer, MS, diabetes, etc., do. Many families that have Lyme in their households struggle on a multitude of levels, with most experiencing significant relational and financial hardships. People with Lyme disease can thus feel isolated, which then causes them to become myopically focused upon Lyme disease alone. It is easy to develop tunnel vision about Borreliosis and co-infections, and forget that most patients with Lyme disease have at least one (and sometimes many) of the co-existing conditions that Connie describes in this book.

Following Connie's suggestions for diagnosis and treatment (with the guidance of a competent Lyme-literate practitioner), should markedly increase the probability of a full recovery from chronic illness, as well as decrease the chances of illness recurrence. Even people who have never had a diagnosis of Borreliosis and/or co-infections but who have Lyme-like symptoms should consider applying the information in this book to resolve their symptoms.

William Lee Cowden, M.D, M.D.(H)

William Lee Cowden, M.D., M.D.(H) graduated from the University of Texas Medical School, in Houston, Texas, and completed residency and fellowship training at St.Louis University Hospital Group. He is US board-certified in cardiology and internal medicine. Early in his career, he recognized the need to focus on the causation of disease, especially chronic disease. He now teaches other health professionals, in person and through The Academy of Comprehensive Integrative Medicine: www.acimconnect.com. While in practice, his focus was on chronic disease of all types. In 2003, he and another doctor conducted a pilot study of Lyme disease that consisted of 27 participants; 14 of whom were in a control group and 13 of whom were in an integrative treatment group. After 70 days, the control group showed minimal to no change in their symptoms, while the 13 in the treatment group all showed marked improvement. Subsequently, in 2007, he worked with Dr. Horowitz in New York State and developed an all-natural treatment program for his chronic Lyme disease patients. As a result of this program, more than 70% of his chronic Lyme patients who had failed pharmaceutical antibiotic therapy improved markedly. Over the years, Dr. Cowden has personally seen many Lyme patients have great success in returning to a "normal" life – including many who had been told by other M.D.s that their cases were hopeless.

A Gift to All Lyme Disease Sufferers

—Marlene E. Kunold

Throughout the centuries, mankind has faced epidemics, some of which erased entire populations of villages, cities, and even countries. The epidemics always occurred for a reason, such as difficult life circumstances, lack of hygiene, no sanitary installations, hunger or cold.

The deep-rooted fear of epidemics throughout history has brought some findings to blossom, and these more or less continue to influence us today.

For instance, the teachings of Louis Pasteur (who was the founder of microbiology) are still being applied today (e.g. pasteurized/heated milk), although Pasteur himself admitted, while dying in 1895, that what he had said during his lifetime was all wrong. It didn´t help to discredit him, as what he taught is still in people's minds and in books today. His famous opponent was French physiologist Claude Bernard, who said: "The microbe is nothing- the terrain (of the body) is everything" (with regards to what determines whether a person will get sick). ("Le germe 'est ien, le terrain est tout!").

The English doctor, Edward Jenner, born in 1749, invented the very first vaccine. It consisted of pus that was taken from a cow that had cowpox, and was thought to be *the* breakthrough in the prevention of small pox. Through this vaccine, Jenner believed that mankind would "win the war" against nature, infection, and mass epidemics.

The idea behind the development of the vaccine was that the body would create immunity when exposed to a small amount of certain microbes. Long-term antibody production would be the aim of the vaccine and also the "proof" of its success.

Vaccinations create high levels of antibodies to the various microbes that are injected into the body, and through them, doctors may prevent acute infections—but for the price of throwing their patients into a chronic state of illness.

Lyme sufferers may know that when their doctors tell them that their Lyme is healed (or in remission), (while looking at blood work which reveals elevated IgG antibodies) that they are really not well. The long-term presence of elevated antibodies generally means that the body is still in a chronic state of infection, and far from being healed or having built up immunity.

Then there are antibiotics, which were first "accidentally" discovered by Alexander Fleming in 1928 in a fungus called Penicillium. It was believed that the antibiotics developed from this fungus would "win the war" against many infections. Equipped with antibiotics and vaccinations—what infection could seriously threaten human health?

The answer is: multiple, chronic, persistant infections, all of which are "embedded" in the various toxic circumstances of modern life.

And, yes, Connie is so right in saying that there is much more to Lyme disease, than just plain infection. Let´s look beyond.

For instance, we are dealing with toxicity from everywhere; all over the planet. Our food is processed and toxic as a result of insecticides, herbicides, food additives, genetic modification, and microwaves. Our meat is loaded with antibiotics, and sugar, sugar, sugar! Our mouths are being "stuffed" with heavy metals from dental amalgams, and dead teeth are being "saved" with root canals.

Modern buildings are a supermarket of toxic fumes. They allow no air to circulate, which creates a favorable environment for mold to grow in. We are silently harming our health.

We love being available to others wherever we go. Radiation from wireless internet connections and cell phones is present everywhere; the TV runs on standby, wireless phones are on at home, and each family member has his or her own computer...and so on. We know today that these pulsed frequencies from radiation tend to disturb endocrine function and sleep/recreational patterns. This can cause adrenal fatigue, immune suppression and "burn out" syndrome.

And, yes, a happy childhood lasts a lifetime. But so does an unhappy one. Childhood, by the way, begins in the mother's uterus. A fetus takes on every single trauma that the pregnant mother goes through. And it takes a certain "behavioral pattern" to attract Lyme disease. If you are not "at home" inside of yourself, the "gangs" (pathogens and xenobiotics) start to hang out in your body... So it's better to "come back home," clean out the filth, and take your space back.

Connie Strasheim, in her book, *Beyond Lyme Disease,* has gone way beyond the average in her look at the Lyme disease situation. She provides a broad look, deep insights, and thorough research into the causes of chronic illness involving Lyme disease.

And there's always more to be learned, as long as you keep your eyes and your mind open. I am sure that Connie will continue to do wonderful research and work that we can all benefit from. This book is a gift to all Lyme disease sufferers, and to all therapists who are truly seeking healing for their patients. She offers various treatment options, and always leaves room for readers to have their own thoughts (come to their own conclusions) and make their own decisions.

Marlene E. Kunold
"Heilpraktiker" (Natural Healing practitioner), Hamburg, Germany

Preface

I was diagnosed with chronic Lyme disease in 2004, more than eight years ago, although my symptoms started several years before that. Since 2004, I have spent most of my days researching medicine, interviewing doctors, helping other people with Lyme disease, and doing treatments to heal from Borreliosis, other Lyme disease-related co-infections, and additional conditions that caused me to become chronically ill. While *Borrelia* and other Lyme disease infections are thought to be principally transmitted through the bite of a tick, some researchers believe that other insects, such as biting flies, mites and mosquitoes, are also vectors for these infections. Mounting evidence indicates that Lyme disease is also spread from human to human via bodily fluids, and from mother to child through the placenta. Studies have proven *Bartonella*, one of the principal Lyme disease infections, to be transmitted through the scratch or bite of a cat. Other mammals, such as squirrels and white-footed mice, also carry the infections, but mainstream research hasn't conclusively proven that the infections can be transmitted to humans through them. For purposes of simplicity, and because *Borrelia* and other Lyme infections are commonly thought to be transmitted through ticks, I will be referring to them as tick-borne infections throughout the book. Please bear in mind, however, that *Borrelia, Babesia, Bartonella, Ehrlichia,* and other commonly recognized Lyme disease infections may also be transmitted through the aforementioned vectors, as well as possibly through others that have yet been unrecognized. Some people with Lyme disease may have never been exposed to ticks or recall a tick bite; however, they may have a spouse with Lyme disease, or have been bitten by a mosquito in a Lyme-endemic region.

Over the years, as a result of interviewing doctors, attending conferences, reading books, researching articles on the Internet, and communicating with countless others who suffer from symptoms of tick-borne infections, I have come to believe that there are two types of people within the Lyme disease community. First, there are those for whom tick-borne infections are the primary instigators of disease and cause of symptoms. These people, when given enough antibiotics or antimicrobial herbal remedies, along with a few detoxification agents or supportive treatments, eventually get better—whether their healing journey takes six months or six years. They heal, if they are working with a good "Lyme-literate" doctor and diligently pursue a comprehensive treatment protocol.

Then there are those for whom tick-borne infections comprise only one component of illness, and that component may be major or minor in the overall symptom picture. The majority of people with chronic Lyme disease fall into this category. Tick-borne infections may or may not have been the instigating factor in their illnesses. Often, the infections simply took advantage of whatever other problems were already going on in the body.

These people either become *more* ill while doing antimicrobial treatments, because they can't effectively detoxify the biotoxins generated by those treatments. Or, they don't progress much in their healing while doing the treatments because the other causes of disease are not being adequately addressed. It is for this group of people that I have written this book.

While some Lyme-literate doctors might agree that all people with Lyme disease need to pursue the strategies in this book (in addition to antimicrobial treatments for tick-borne infections), not all would agree that the causes of disease mentioned here are the primary instigators of illness in people with Lyme. My research and experiences have taught me however, that other factors cause disease in people with Lyme. These factors can be just as, if not more, significant than tick-borne infections. Thus, it's important to discuss them at length, so that people with Lyme and their doctors give them the attention they deserve, rather than simply regarding them as ancillary conditions that result from Lyme.

Discerning the root causes of illness in people with tick-borne infections is somewhat of a "chicken and egg" game, since it can be difficult to know which disease processes trigger symptoms. For instance, adrenal fatigue, one of the topics addressed in this book, can be a cause or result of illness from tick-borne infections. Gastrointestinal problems can result from tick-borne infections, but they can also cause the body to become susceptible to infections. This book describes conditions that are both causes and effects of tick-borne illness, but its focus is upon how to treat them, as if they were primary causes of disease.

Some people may argue that it's irrelevant which came first—the chicken or the egg—because all of the conditions and symptoms that are found in people with chronic Lyme disease must be treated. I have learned, however, that whatever is assumed to be the primary cause of disease—tick-borne infections, for instance—tends to become the focus of treatment, and less attention is given to the management of other conditions. In other words, emphasis is placed upon treating infections, when in reality treatment should focus equally upon other major causes of illness.

I wrote this book because I have observed that in general, the Lyme disease community has focused mostly upon treating tick-borne infections, when other conditions are often the main cause of their woes. My hope in this book is to encourage people with Lyme, and their doctors, to consider what else might be causing symptoms besides infections, especially when antibiotic or other treatments for tick-borne infections have proven to be insufficient for healing.

Chronic illness involving Lyme disease is a quagmire for even the most brilliant minds. No Lyme-literate physician or practitioner who treats chronic illness has a perfect track record with patients, because no treatment works on 100 percent of the people, 100 percent of the time. But some people aren't getting better because their doctors are focusing mostly upon tick-borne infections, when in truth, multiple factors are conspiring to make them sick, and some of these factors are just as, if not more, important than the infections.

If you opened this book hoping to find information on antimicrobial treatments for some of the most important tick-borne infections, such as *Borrelia burgdorferi* (and the other dozens of *Borrelias*), *Babesia* (babesiosis), *Bartonella, Ehrlichia* and others, you won't find an in-depth analysis about those here. I do briefly describe some of the latest treatments for tick-borne infections, according to Lyme-literate doctors, in the Appendix. Also, consider my book *Insights into Lyme Disease Treatment: 13 Lyme-Literate Health Care Practitioners Share Their Healing Strategies* (www.lymeinsights. com) for a more in-depth look at how to treat tick-borne infections using antibiotics, herbs, and holistic medicine.

What you will find here are insights into what is making thousands of people in the United States and around the world sick. It's not just tick-borne infections; it's tick-borne infections along with a plethora of environmental toxins and other factors. While this book is written for those who have been diagnosed with Lyme disease, the topics are relevant for anyone suffering from symptoms of environmental illness or symptoms and conditions that mimic Lyme disease.

These symptoms include, but are not limited to:

- Chronic fatigue syndrome
- Fibromyalgia
- Lupus
- Arthritis
- Multiple chemical sensitivities
- Allergies
- Multiple sclerosis
- ALS
- Parkinson's

Disease labels sometimes matter anyway in complex illnesses involving multiple body systems and organs. Becoming fixated on a single diagnosis can blind people to other problems that might be underlying their symptoms.

Regardless of the instigating factors of disease, however, once the body falls apart, treating the instigating factors alone becomes insufficient for healing. By the time symptoms appear, many things have gone wrong bio-chemically. Healing the body requires addressing systemic dysfunction on multiple levels, so that the body can be restored little by little. Fortunately, some open-minded healthcare practitioners who continually research the latest advances in alternative and integrative medicine are coming up with better solutions for complex illness involving Lyme disease, environmental illness, and other conditions that mimic Lyme, such as chronic fatigue syndrome and fibromyalgia. With proper attention to their causes, great strides can be made in healing.

Finally, while the conditions described in this book represent some of the most important causes of sickness in people with tick-borne infections, the book does not mention every principal cause of illness in people with Lyme. I describe only those that I know about and which contribute to illness in a majority of people. Also, this work is not meant to provide in-depth treatment information for every condition. For that, I recommend consulting a healthcare practitioner who specializes in the conditions described herein, as well as doing further research on the topics.

I hope that my insights, experience, and knowledge will be a source of encouragement and hope to those seeking to heal from chronic illness involving Lyme, especially those who haven't experienced significant improvements in their well-being—despite years of antibiotics or antimi-crobial treatments. I also hope that this work will provide insights to Lyme-literate doctors and other healthcare practitioners who have learned that effectively treating patients involves much more than simply addressing tick-borne infections; it involves treating every underlying cause of disease that is contributing to symptoms.

Chapter One

Adrenal Insufficiency and Hypothyroidism

The adrenal glands play an extremely important role in the body. They are, first and foremost, involved in immune function and the body's stress response. They also regulate blood sugar levels, blood pressure, inflammation, blood vessel constriction, and electrolyte balance in the cells, among other things. They help mobilize protein for energy use by the body, and aid in carrying thyroid hormones from the blood to the cells.

Adrenal insufficiency is a condition in which the adrenal glands fail to produce proper amounts of steroid hormones and adrenalin, which are used by the body for all of the aforementioned processes. The condition is due to prolonged stress from disease, trauma, or toxins. Sometimes it is caused by adrenals that are inherently weak.

Based on my research and experience, I believe that adrenal fatigue is a principal, or triggering cause of illness in many people with tick-borne infections, chronic fatigue syndrome, and other conditions involving severe autonomic nervous system dysfunction. Adrenal insufficiency can cause detoxification problems, postural orthostatic tachycardia syndrome, dysautonomias, and other neuroendocrine problems (which are usually attributed to the effects of tick-borne infections). Adrenal insufficiency can be caused by tick-borne infections, but it can also be what triggers tick-borne illness. Since it is usually assumed to be a result of Lyme disease, in this chapter, I will focus on why it is also often a cause.

Adrenal Fatigue Symptoms

Below is a list of common adrenal fatigue symptoms. Most of these overlap with symptoms of chronic Lyme disease. Since chronic Lyme disease causes adrenal fatigue, it can be difficult to judge the primary cause of symptoms in a person with Lyme. Yet the primary cause of symptoms is important to know, for reasons that I will explain subsequently.

- Chronic fatigue
- Musculoskeletal pain
- Anxiety
- Depression
- Feeling "wired but tired"
- Needing to sleep more than eight hours per night
- Being tired in the morning, and awake at night
- Insomnia
- Irritable bowel syndrome
- Hypotension (low blood pressure)
- Environmental and food allergies
- Hypoglycemia (low blood sugar)
- Nervousness
- Sensitivity to sounds/light
- Irritability
- Feeling easily agitated by life's stressors
- Multiple chemical sensitivities
- Food allergies
- Loss of libido
- Low body temperature
- Low energy
- Menstrual irregularities and PMS
- Heart palpitations
- Sugar and salt cravings
- Postural orthostatic tachycardia syndrome

Causes of Adrenal Fatigue

Infections weaken the adrenal glands, but so do many other stressors, including sugar, caffeine, alcohol, allergenic foods, environmental toxins, and, especially, emotional stress. Some people have a genetic predisposition to adrenal fatigue. It is often found in people who are tall, slender, sensitive, and intuitive.

The late Gerald Poesnecker, ND worked with adrenally fatigued patients for over forty years. He authored the book *Chronic Fatigue Unmasked.* Dr. Poesnecker found adrenal insufficiency to be a primary cause of chronic fatigue syndrome and other health conditions in many of his patients. In the introduction to his book, he wrote, "I feel that Chronic Fatigue Syndrome, as usually diagnosed, is usually identical with Adrenal Syndrome, and that these two conditions are caused by a gradual accumulation of small, but potent stresses that eventually create an overload of the immune system that the traditional prescription of time and rest is inadequate to correct."

In his more than four decades of work with patients, he discerned that most of his adrenal patients were sensitive and intuitive, with tendencies to overwork and take on too many burdens—conditions that triggered and/or perpetuated the problem. I have observed that living in fear, perfectionism, and "fast-forward" mode are also characteristics that can cause or perpetuate adrenal fatigue. People with weak constitutions also tend to have weak adrenal glands.

Dr. Poesnecker hasn't been the only practitioner to believe in adrenal fatigue as a primary cause of disease. Michael Lam, MD, on his website www.drlam. com, writes that many experts believe that adrenal fatigue precedes chronic fatigue syndrome and fibromyalgia. It causes the dysfunction of multiple organs and bodily systems, which leads to a multitude of problems.

Because the adrenal glands are strongly involved in immune function, people with adrenal insufficiency constantly battle infections. Their bodies are easily affected by stressors, from allergenic foods to financial woes to bad relationships. Tick-borne infections are part of their stressor package. While eliminating the infections may relieve some of the stress that has been placed upon their adrenal glands, if adrenal dysfunction preceded their infections, getting rid of these infections may be insufficient for their recovery. Further, many will not be able to eliminate the infections, because their adrenal insufficiency hasn't been adequately treated. Their bodies can't mount an effective immune response against the infections.

Scientific studies have proven that when the body is in a constant state of stress, its "fight or flight response" sympathetic nervous system is activated. This causes the adrenal glands to release high amounts of cortisol and adrenaline. If the response is chronic and prolonged, it weakens the adrenal glands and disables the immune system, allowing pathogens to flourish and toxins to accumulate in the body.

In addition to having a constitutional (genetic) or character predisposition to the condition, many people with adrenal insufficiency have either suffered from abuse or experienced many severe stressful events over their lifetime. Numerous studies have established that trauma plays a significant role in the development of chronic illness, especially in women. Female biochemistry tends to be more significantly altered by emotional trauma than male biochemistry.

In any case, the root cause of disease in people who have severe adrenal fatigue and Lyme isn't always tick-borne infections. The infections are simply one manifestation of a suppressed immune system caused by adrenal dysfunction, but their presence exacerbates the adrenal dysfunction. Therefore, healing requires placing a strong emphasis upon healing the adrenals, along with treating the infections. Because symptoms of adrenal fatigue overlap with those of chronic Lyme disease, and Lyme disease causes adrenal fatigue, it can be difficult to discern how much emphasis to place upon treating adrenal fatigue. A strong, supportive protocol for the adrenal glands must be undertaken, along with antimicrobial treatments, when adrenal fatigue precedes Lyme or is heavily implicated in the Lyme disease symptom picture. Extremely aggressive antimicrobial protocols can also make people with adrenal fatigue worse. Later in this chapter, I describe some treatments that are effective for healing the adrenal glands.

My Story of Adrenal Fatigue

I am passionate about the topic of adrenal insufficiency because I believe that it was a primary cause of my symptoms, along with tick-borne infections. I have suffered from symptoms of adrenal fatigue throughout my life, even for many years prior to becoming infected by a tick. Such symptoms have included moderate fatigue, back pain, brain fog, anxiety, hypoglycemia, and the phenomenon of being "wired yet tired." I have always had more energy at night, and needed excessive amounts of sleep. My physical constitution, temperament, and character also fit the typical "adrenal fatigue profile," which has been described by adrenal fatigue experts such as Dr. Poesnecker. And over the years, as I have studied adrenal fatigue and other disease conditions, and monitored my symptoms, I have discerned adrenal fatigue to be one of the main conditions that set the stage for me to become ill from tick-borne and other infections. The infections simply took advantage of a weakened immune system caused by adrenal fatigue.

I received treatment for tick-borne infections and environmental toxicity for approximately six years, and I believe that this was crucial for my healing. Infections and toxins cause serious damage to the body and must be eliminated. Yet eliminating infections and environmental toxins only minimally mitigated my symptoms. On the other hand, I have always experienced radical improvements to my well-being whenever I have focused upon healing my adrenals, rather than attacking infections (regardless of how long I treated the infections). I have also seldom experienced severe Herxheimer reactions as a result of aggressive antimicrobial treatments, or such treatments would cause me to have extremely prolonged Herxheimer reactions (which can indicate detoxification problems caused by adrenal insufficiency). For this and other reasons, I believe that tick-borne infections were a secondary cause of my symptoms, and that the primary cause was immune dysfunction caused by weak adrenals.

I have communicated with other people with Lyme disease who also believe that their symptoms were directly caused by adrenal insufficiency and that this set the stage for them to become ill from tick-borne infections. These people say that treatments for tick-borne infections either made them worse or were only minimally helpful. One wonderful lady who suffers from Lyme disease, Anne Davis, in a personal message to me on October 8, 2011, wrote that she believed she would have had better outcomes with her Lyme treatments if she had been treated for adrenal insufficiency first. She wrote:

"In 2007, when I was finally diagnosed with chronic Lyme disease, I began treatments for Borrelia and Bartonella. And then once we started, and realized I had Babesia, all hell broke loose. I only did oral antibiotics/malaria meds . . . no IV . . . . In hindsight, I think I would have done much better if I hadn't been dealing with a genetic detoxification issue; if we wouldn't have busted up biofilms way too quickly; if we would have gone much slower on killing everything off; if my severe adrenal fatigue had been addressed first (but my LLMD [Lyme-literate medical doctor] didn't know that this was why my thyroid [hormone levels] were scary rock-bottom low)." Later in the message, she adds, "I really wish LLMDs knew much more about detoxification/nutritional support/addressing severe adrenal fatigue [instead of just addressing the thyroid]—things that LLMDs seem to know best . . . I know more people [including myself], who are working with an LLMD and an LLND . . . . So many people have severe adrenal fatigue, and I've heard so many stories about LLMDs putting them on blood pressure meds, because their blood pressure is so low—instead of addressing the low [dysfunctional] adrenals. They just don't know [that this is a major problem in people with Lyme disease]."

Treating Adrenal Insufficiency/Dysfunction

Healing from adrenal fatigue is tricky, because unlike infections or environmental toxins, simply taking a few remedies or toxin binders won't fix the problem. While adrenal-support remedies are helpful, they are usually insufficient by themselves. Adrenal dysfunction represents, at its core, an accumulation or mishandling of life's stressors, on multiple levels. Yes, it is often the result of infections and environmental toxins, but it's also the result of trauma, overworking, perfectionism, rushing through life, self-destructive behaviors, isolation, a poor diet, an inability to set healthy boundaries with people, and operating out of fear rather than trust.

Some people may have been born with a genetic predisposition to adrenal fatigue. Because the adrenal glands handle the body's response to stressors of all kinds, healing them requires addressing all of the factors that caused the adrenal glands and the immune system to become weak in the first place. For some people, healing requires an entire revamping and restructuring of the way they think about, and "do," life. Obviously, it's not all about the Lyme infections.

While a proposition of this kind may seem overwhelming, addressing the root causes of adrenal dysfunction will render infectious and other causes of disease less important and easier to treat. It will also keep the body, spirit, and soul healthier over the long haul. It's important to note, however, that once infections are causing symptoms in the body, they must also be treated, along with the adrenal glands.

Whenever I have had the discipline, I have followed Dr. Lam's website and personal recommendations for treating adrenal fatigue, and always experienced improvements to my overall well-being. I say, "whenever I have had the discipline," because healing the adrenals is a multifaceted endeavor that requires discipline and a strong desire to get well, and most people (including me) can't eliminate all stressful or self-sabotaging behavior from their lives in order to fully heal. Hence the need for self-control and a powerful will to get well. At the same time, treatments in themselves can be a major source of stress, so doing what you can while accepting that you can't do everything right is probably a better approach than trying to be perfect, since perfectionism perpetuates the condition.

Strategies for reducing or eliminating the emotional and lifestyle stressors that contribute to adrenal fatigue are described in Chapter Eight. For a more comprehensive look at how to heal adrenal fatigue, I recommend reading books devoted exclusively to the subject, some of which are recommended in the References and Resources section at the end of this book. I especially recommend Dr. Lam's recently-released *Adrenal Fatigue Syndrome,* which provides an in-depth look at the causes of adrenal fatigue, the metabolic and other systemic dysfunctions that are created by adrenal fatigue, as well as treatments for the condition. For anyone wanting to learn more about this subject, this book is an essential resource.

In general, strategies for healing the adrenal glands include learning how to move through life with a sense of trust rather than fear, eliminating abusive relationships, learning to set healthy relational boundaries with others, getting involved in life, learning to rest, having down time every day, living at a sane pace, eating well, eliminating workaholism, avoiding negative chatter, getting enough sleep at night, and healing past traumas that contribute to fearful, angry thinking and behaviors. Many supplements and other remedies can also aid recovery. By themselves, they are insufficient for most people who suffer from moderately severe or severe adrenal fatigue, but they are an essential adjunct to lifestyle strategies for healing.

Unfortunately, confusion abounds in the medical field over the best way to treat adrenal dysfunction or insufficiency. There is also no such thing as a "one size fits all" approach to adrenal support. Adrenal supplements need to be prescribed according to individual biochemistry and the severity of the adrenal fatigue. Adrenal supplements are often misused and improperly prescribed because these factors aren't taken into account. For example, in the concluding remarks of his article "Adrenal Fatigue Glandular and Herbal Therapy," Dr. Lam writes:

> "Herbs and glandulars are widely used and touted as possessing adaptogenic properties and marketed as tonics. They are popular with those with very mild Adrenal Fatigue, due to their stimulatory properties [which] increase energy and reduce fatigue. These stimulatory effects are more pronounced, the weaker the adrenals. [But] stimulants are the equivalent of giving too much gas and "flooding the engine" in a car. They put further stress on the adrenals to work harder and produce more energy, and end up further depleting the adrenal glands. While there may be short-term benefits [from them], this often produces a false sense of well-being that over time tends to fail."

Some of the herbal remedies that Dr. Lam notes as being potentially too stimulatory for those with adrenal fatigue include: Siberian ginseng, ashwagandha root, Panax ginseng, and licorice root. According to Dr. Lam, and depending upon how these herbs are used, they may increase stamina and decrease symptoms in the short run, but over the long haul, they can exhaust the adrenal glands even more. Dr. Lam also writes:

> "While the use of glandulars and herbs have their places in adrenal recovery, their use must be judicious to avoid overstimulation,

addiction, and withdrawal concerns. Short-term use in very mild cases [of adrenal fatigue] is acceptable, but it is best to proceed under the supervision of an experienced adrenal expert if adrenal weakness is pronounced. Always be on the alert [for] paradoxical or unusual reactions (such as excessive stimulation, excessive fatigue, cardiac palpitation, unstable blood pressure, insomnia, anxiety, and irritability) as warning signs of inappropriate use. . . ."

I received over-the-phone counsel from Dr. Lam for several months for my own case of adrenal fatigue and learned that taking too many supplements simultaneously also stresses the adrenal glands. The body has to break down and either utilize or discard the constituents of all those supplements, which takes energy. If you suffer from severe adrenal fatigue, taking a few well-selected remedies may be better than taking ten or twenty supplements every day. Because Dr. Lam diagnosed me as having severe adrenal fatigue, his protocol for me involved taking no herbal remedies, because he believed that these would be too stimulatory for my body. Instead, he prescribed nutrients to rebuild my adrenals, and an all-natural, low-glycemic diet, free of refined sugar, preservatives, additives, dairy and other inflammatory foods.

Following are some of the most all-around effective nutrients/supplements for treating adrenal fatigue. Most people with moderate to severe adrenal fatigue can safely benefit from these.

Liposomal Vitamin C

Vitamin C regenerates the adrenal glands. Most of the body's vitamin C is utilized by the adrenals. Many vitamin C products, such as plain ascorbic acid, are ineffective and manufactured in a form that the body cannot use (they are also often corn-based, and many people with Lyme disease are allergic to corn). Liposomal nutrients, which are encased in fat, tend to be better absorbed by the body. People with severe adrenal fatigue should start on a low dose of liposomal vitamin C, around 500 mg, and work up to 2,000 mg or more per day if continual improvements are felt and they don't "crash" on increased doses. Pure Horizon makes a tasty, effective liposomal vitamin C product called LipoNano C, which can be purchased at Supplement Clinic (www.supplementclinic.com).

Pantethine

This is a highly bioavailable metabolite of pantothenic acid, which also helps to rebuild the adrenal glands. People with severe adrenal fatigue should start out on a low dose and build up slowly. Dr. Lam prescribed a product called Pandrenal (also made by Pure Horizon) to me. I took three 300 mg capsules, twice daily.

Liposomal Glutathione

Glutathione is an important antioxidant involved in detoxification. When the adrenals are fatigued, the body's ability to produce glutathione is compromised. Glutathione acts as a potent liver detoxifier and helps to recycle inactive oxidized vitamin C back to an active form, once it has served its function in the body. Dr. Lam prescribed 2 tsp/day of a product called LipoNano Glutathione for me. As with LipoNano C and Pandrenal, LipoNano Glutathione may be purchased at Supplement Clinic: www.supplementclinic.com.

Note: While I believe the aforementioned remedies could be effective remedies for many with advanced adrenal fatigue, I recommend consulting Dr. Lam or another hormone specialist for a customized treatment regimen. Also, I receive no financial incentive from Pure Horizon, Supplement Clinic, or any of Dr. Lam's recommended product suppliers for the promotion of their products.

Amino Acids

Amino acids are the building blocks of protein from which all tissue is made, and thus give our body substance. The proper proportion of a variety of amino acids helps to rebuild and regenerate exhausted adrenals. Dr. Lam prescribes an amino acid product called Quantum to some of his patients for this purpose. This product may also be found at Supplement Clinic: www.supplementclinic.com.

Finally, freshly prepared chicken broth (not from a can or box) is very healing to the adrenal glands. Chicken bones and cartilage contain powerful substances that rebuild and strengthen adrenals. Drinking two to four cups daily is an important component of the adrenal regeneration process. The fresher the chicken broth, the better.

People who suffer from severe adrenal fatigue may also require a prescription of hydrocortisone and/or fludrocortisone (if aldosterone levels are also low), but these are most often prescribed temporarily. Some doctors don't advocate their use unless absolutely necessary. Supplemental steroid hormones are thought to give the adrenals a rest, so that they don't have to produce as much of their own hormones. The hormones do this by replacing deficient levels of cortisol and aldosterone in the body. They do not, however, rebuild the adrenals. They should be taken in conjunction with a comprehensive adrenal-healing protocol.

That said, Dr. Lam writes on his website: www.drlam.com, that when hormonal homeostasis is severely disturbed, steroid hormone replacement, as well as adrenal glandular formulas, can make some people with severe adrenal fatigue feel worse instead of better. And steroids such as hydrocortisone aren't without long-term side effects. Studies indicate that the adrenal glands can become dependent upon them, especially at higher doses. The consensus in the medical community, which seems to be based largely upon information found in the book *Safe Uses of Cortisol* by Jeffrey Bland, MD, is that hydrocortisone dosages of up to 20 mg daily are safe. My belief is that as all things in medicine, it depends upon the person. The medical community needs to learn more about the endocrine system before it can come to definitive conclusions about the safety of supplemental steroid hormones.

Debate continues within the medical community over whether steroid use, particularly hydrocortisone, is safe for people with chronic Lyme disease. Some doctors believe that if cortisol levels are lower than what they should be, bringing them to normal levels with physiological doses of supplemental hydrocortisone shouldn't cause immune suppression. That it should, in fact, support immune function, because not having enough cortisol in the body is just as detrimental as having too much. Others say that people with Lyme disease should not, under any circumstances, take steroid hormones, since these can cause infections to flare. Whether or not this is true probably depends upon the person and amount of steroid hormone that is taken. Some people with Lyme disease have become irrevocably sicker after taking steroid hormones. Doctors should consider very carefully whether to prescribe them to their patients.

The Adrenal Diet

Besides taking supplements, maintaining a proper diet is important for healing from adrenal fatigue. Any food that is inflammatory or allergenic will stress the adrenals. One of the functions of the adrenal glands is to release cortisol, to mediate the inflammatory response caused by allergenic foods. Caffeinated beverages and refined sugar are perhaps the biggest adrenal stressors. Other inflammatory agents include many grains and all pasteurized dairy, along with all genetically-modified non-organic and processed foods containing additives. More about the kind of diet that I recommend for people with chronic illness involving Lyme is discussed in Chapter Two. It's important to remove all sources of inflammation from the body in order to heal the adrenal glands, including inflammation which is caused by unhealthy and allergenic food.

Eating small, frequent meals that include animal protein, healthy fats such as olive and coconut oil, and low-glycemic carbohydrates reduces adrenal stress and helps to combat the hypoglycemia that often accompanies adrenal fatigue. Skipping meals or eating large meals stresses the adrenals. Having a small amount of animal protein or some nuts before bedtime is also essential, as it helps to stabilize blood sugar levels during the night. Cooked stews and soups, filled with non-starchy vegetables and animal protein, are good meal choices for the adrenally fatigued. They stabilize blood sugar and are easy to digest. While some healthcare practitioners advocate eating high quantities of raw vegetables, people with adrenal fatigue tend to have low levels of stomach acid and cannot easily digest raw veggies. A combination of raw and cooked vegetables is probably better for most.

For more information on how to treat adrenal fatigue, please see the References and Resources section at the end of this book.

Diagnosing Adrenal Fatigue

A diagnosis of adrenal fatigue or insufficiency should be primarily based upon symptoms, along with lab test results. However, many lab tests are inaccurate, which is why working with a doctor who understands the condition and can diagnose it by analyzing symptoms is important.

The most reliable lab test is a 24-hour saliva cortisol test, which measures the amount of free-circulating cortisol and other adrenal hormones. Practitioners who prescribe this test for their patients should be aware that some people can have test results that fall within the "normal" range and yet be symptomatic, while others may display few symptoms but have abnormal lab test results. This is because the range of what is considered to be normal varies from person to person. However, saliva cortisol tests can provide helpful insights about the severity of the adrenal insufficiency. For more information about how to accurately evaluate steroid hormone levels, especially cortisol, I recommend Janie Bowthorpe's book, *Stop the Thyroid Madness*.

The Problem with High-Dose Antibiotic Protocols for People with Adrenal Fatigue

Many Lyme-literate doctors contend that high-dose antibiotic and herbal protocols are necessary to eliminate tick-borne infections. These protocols usually involve taking high doses of multiple antibiotics or antimicrobial substances, often intravenously, for many months, several years, or indefinitely. Pharmaceutical antibiotics not only deplete the body of healthy bacteria, especially in the gastrointestinal tract, but also stress the organs, including the adrenal glands. As the body eliminates neurotoxins generated by infectious-organism die-off, the adrenals are further taxed, since they play an important role in detoxification.

Of course, reducing the body's infection load removes stress from the adrenals over the long run, which is a good thing. But it is a bit of a catch-22, since treating infections too aggressively can stress the adrenal glands to the point of making a person worse instead of better. While it may be necessary to use aggressive doses of medications to get rid of infections, doctors need to be careful to not exhaust their patients' adrenals beyond their capacity to help the body to recover from Lyme. Besides Anne Davis, who was mentioned earlier in this chapter, I have spoken with dozens of people who, instead of improving, suffered an exacerbation of their symptoms after aggressive and prolonged antibiotic regimens. I believe that for some, this happened because their adrenal glands weren't adequately supported during treatment, or their treatment regimens were too aggressive. I have also spoken with several Lyme-literate healthcare practitioners such as Marlene Kunold, a "Heilpraktiker" (health practitioner) in Germany, who contends that some will get worse on aggressive treatment regiments unless their adrenals are strongly supported.

Some people get worse on antibiotic protocols for tick-borne infections because they stop their regimens prematurely, take inappropriate combinations of antimicrobial medications at the wrong doses, or don't support their bodies' detoxification processes. Other people's glandular systems become overwhelmed by treatments. As a result, they are unable to mount a sufficient immune response against the infections. Still others may not be able to eliminate the toxins generated by infections, which again, can be due in part to adrenal insufficiency, since the adrenals aid in detoxification. Everyone who battles tick-borne infections suffers from some degree of adrenal stress. Yet those who had adrenal fatigue prior to getting *Borreliosis* and co-infections, may struggle more in their recovery, and even get worse on strong antimicrobial regimens.

Steven Bock, MD, in my book *Insights into Lyme Disease Treatment,* describes how he bases his treatments upon concepts found in Chinese medicine, which recognizes that people have varying constitutions and, therefore, require different treatments. People who are more "yin," for example, tend to have weaker adrenal glands and may require a gentler approach to treatment. While many Lyme-literate doctors believe that an aggressive treatment approach is necessary for eliminating tick-borne infections, the situation is challenging for those with weak adrenal glands. A less-aggressive protocol that involves strong support for the adrenals may be more beneficial, depending upon whether aggressive treatments seem to produce no improvement after many months, or the body becomes severely weakened by them.

The Link between Adrenal Insufficiency and Hypothyroidism

Adrenal insufficiency affects thyroid hormone uptake and utilization and causes hypothyroidism. The thyroid gland supplies hormones to keep the metabolism in working order. Hypothyroidism is a condition in which the thyroid gland is either not functioning properly and is producing suboptimal levels of thyroid hormones, or the body isn't utilizing those hormones properly. In the case of adrenal fatigue, hypothyroidism is caused by the latter condition. This is important to know because when thyroid hormone uptake and utilization have been affected by adrenal fatigue, both the thyroid and adrenals must be treated in order for a full recovery to occur.

Hypothyroidism is common in people with chronic illnesses such as Lyme disease, fibromyalgia, and chronic fatigue syndrome, and can be a major cause of symptoms in people with tick-borne infections. Often it occurs concurrently with adrenal insufficiency and is a direct result of it. Dr. Lam writes on his website (www.drlam.com): "Adrenal Fatigue is perhaps the most common cause of secondary low thyroid function, both clinically and sub-clinically. Low adrenal function often leads to low thyroid function, [which is] classically evidenced by high levels of thyroid binding globulin (a protein used to carry T4 and T3 in the bloodstream), low free T4, low free T3, high TSH, slow ankle reflex and low body temperature."

When the adrenals are exhausted, their ability to handle the stress of normal bodily functions and the body's energy requirements becomes compromised. In response to this, the body lowers its metabolic rate and energy output by down-regulating the thyroid function. This gives the adrenal glands an opportunity to rest and recover, since lower energy output and a slower metabolism means that they don't have to work as hard to function. As the thyroid down-regulates its functioning, it decreases its production of T4 and T3 hormones. T4 is an inactive form of thyroid hormone, which the body converts to T3, the body's most abundant and active form of thyroid hormone. When the adrenal glands are fatigued, the body also shuttles some of its available T4 toward the production of reverse T3 (rT3), another inactive form of thyroid hormone, which opposes and limits the function of active T3. Thus, rT3 causes the body to slow down its metabolic activity by lowering the amount of T3 that is usable by the body and also inhibits the conversion of T4 to T3. This means that if adrenal fatigue is a primary cause of hypothyroidism, taking supplemental T4 hormone can worsen symptoms, since the body will tend to make rT3 from that T4 (instead of active T3), which then reduces the activity of whatever active thyroid hormone (T3) is already in the bloodstream! For this reason, people with moderate to severe adrenal fatigue often feel better by taking supplemental bioidentical T3 hormone, without any T4 added to the mix.

Adrenal insufficiency often results in hypothyroid symptoms and is the true cause of hypothyroidism in many with chronic illness involving Lyme disease. Unfortunately, many healthcare practitioners don't realize that adrenal fatigue is the primary reason for their chronically ill patients' hypothyroidism. By giving them supplemental thyroid hormone without treating their adrenal glands, they are actually making the problem worse. They are forcing the body to increase its metabolic rate, when what it really needs is to slow down, so that the adrenals, which play a vital role in immune function, can recover. As I previously mentioned, whenever adrenal insufficiency is a primary cause of hypothyroidism, both the adrenal insufficiency and hypothyroidism must be treated.

Some healthcare practitioners prescribe their adrenally fatigued and hypothyroid patients supplemental thyroid hormones (both T4 and T3, or just one or the other), along with adrenal gland nutrients and supportive herbal supplements. If only the thyroid is treated, and/or the adrenals aren't adequately supported, the body will continue to down-regulate its thyroid activity as the adrenals become increasingly exhausted. Over time, patients will need increasingly higher amounts of supplemental thyroid hormone in order to effectively treat their symptoms, as their adrenals become more and more depleted.

Janie Bowthorpe, medical researcher and author of the book *Stop the Thyroid Madness,* believes that physiological doses of supplemental steroid hormones, especially the principal adrenal steroid hormone cortisol, are needed to heal the adrenals when they are severely depleted. She contends that natural treatments are likely to be insufficient. Because some people have problems absorbing supplemental cortisol, she notes that physiological doses for some may be as high as 40 mg/day, because not all of that will be absorbed and effectively utilized by the body. She contends that it is rare for someone to need doses that high. However, she has observed that most people need doses of 20–30 mg to feel better over the long haul.

Finding smart solutions to normalize both thyroid and adrenal gland function is vital for healing from chronic illness. For mild to moderate cases of adrenal fatigue, adrenal nutrients may be sufficient for healing, when given in conjunction with thyroid hormone precursors, such as iodine and L-tyrosine, or low doses of bioidentical T3. But for moderate to severe adrenal fatigue, which is most often the case for people with chronic illness, supplemental adrenal steroid hormones may need to be given in conjunction with moderate doses of bioidentical thyroid hormones. Adrenal nutrients such as Vitamin C and pantothenic acid (or pantethine) are effective for rebuilding burned-out adrenals, but their immediate effects upon the body are not as powerful as those experienced with adrenal steroid hormones such as cortisol and aldosterone. If doctors give their patients thyroid hormones without also giving them supplemental adrenal hormones (especially cortisol), it may put additional demands upon the adrenals to function and hinder their ability to recover.

Compromised adrenal function and the resulting compromised thyroid function will effectively prevent healing from Lyme disease—and cause many other problems.

Please bear in mind, my hypotheses and recommendations are based upon my experience and what I have learned from experts about adrenal fatigue and thyroid function. They are not based on double-blind, placebo-controlled trials or thousands of clinical outcome studies (which also have their limitations). I caution readers to not take my contentions as undisputed fact nor as the final authoritative word on thyroid/adrenal hormone treatment.

Many people with Lyme and other chronic illnesses pay attention to and support their adrenal glands, but their adrenals still fail to recover. This may be because they are constantly pushing them beyond their comfort level by taking supplemental thyroid hormones without also undertaking a comparatively strong adrenal regimen to compensate for the increased thyroid metabolism. It may also be that their adrenal function remains compromised due to infections, toxins, and other stressors. If they are able to remove these factors, they may be better equipped to tolerate supplemental thyroid hormone therapy.

All this said, doctors don't generally advocate taking adrenal steroid hormones for long periods of time because they are thought to shut down the body's own production of adrenal hormones. Over time, a person's immune function can be suppressed if the person is improperly dosed. Dr. McJefferies, in his book *Safe Uses of Cortisol*, contends that supplemental cortisol, at physiological doses of 20 mg or less daily, is safe for most people, but that higher doses will cause irreversible suppression of adrenal gland hormone production. Other physicians believe that even lower doses of cortisol, when taken for extended periods of time, can cause this problem. In any case, supplemental cortisol does not always improve symptoms.

Janie Bowthorpe, in her book *Stop the Thyroid Madness*, writes that some people can feel poorly on low doses of hydrocortisone, for different reasons. Sometimes, for instance, the adrenal glands will perceive the presence of the supplemental hormone in the body and shut down their own production of steroid hormones, which results in an even greater deficiency of cortisol and an exacerbation of symptoms. Bowthorpe contends that this adrenal suppression also happens when people take higher doses of steroid hormones, but that higher doses of steroids can compensate for what the body stops making when it senses the presence of the supplemental hormones. Bowthorpe has observed that people often require doses of at least 20 mg of cortisol daily to compensate for what the body stops making. She cautions those who are already taking thyroid hormone to temporarily decrease their thyroid hormone dosage when starting supplemental cortisol, or they may experience surges of adrenaline. This occurs as a result of the body uptaking massive amounts of T3 from the blood, which it was previously unable to utilize, since cortisol aids in thyroid hormone utilization. For more information about the relationship between thyroid and adrenal hormones, I highly recommend reading Bowthorpe's book.

The issue of thyroid and adrenal treatment is a complicated one, and there are no definitive solutions for how to best concurrently treat adrenal and thyroid dysfunction. I'm not convinced that taking 20 mg or more of supplemental hydrocortisone daily is wise for people with chronic Lyme disease since there has been evidence that steroid use causes infections to flare; however, this may be because patients have typically been prescribed doses that exceed their bodies' normal cortisol production levels. At the same time, I don't believe that it is wise for people whose hypothyroidism is caused by adrenal insufficiency to take high doses of supplemental thyroid hormone if they don't also strongly support their adrenal glands. Natural remedies for the adrenals may or may not be sufficient for this purpose. I would simply encourage people who have been diagnosed with hypo-thyroidism to consider adrenal insufficiency as a primary cause of their hypothyroidism, and to take steps to strongly support their adrenals before attempting to put together a treatment protocol for the thyroid.

Regardless of whether adrenal insufficiency is a primary cause of hypo-roidism, hypothyroidism must be corrected, because the thyroid is respon-sible for a plethora of metabolic processes in the body. Hypothyroidism can cause a myriad of symptoms, including fatigue, depression, brain fog, insomnia, and weight gain. Healing from chronic illness is difficult if the thyroid isn't functioning optimally.

Testing Thyroid Function

Most generic TSH tests are inadequate for diagnosing hypothyroidism. Practitioners should order lab panels that measure total TSH, free T3, free and total T4, and reverse T3, along with antibody tests to rule out autoim-mune thyroid ("Hashimoto's") disease.

As previously noted, high levels of reverse T3, an inactive form of thyroid hormone, counteract active thyroid hormone (T3) and prevent it from being effectively utilized by the body. Usually, even free T3 levels that are on the low end of the "normal" range indicate hypothyroidism, although if severe adrenal fatigue is also present, the body's free T3 levels will be falsely elevated, since the body isn't making enough cortisol to effectively uptake thyroid hormone from the blood into the cells (thus, high levels of thyroid hormone remain in the blood and distort test results). The British physician Barry Durrant-Peatfield, in his book *Your Thyroid and How to Keep It Healthy,* contends that some people have high blood levels of thyroid hormone because their cells aren't effectively utilizing it, due to low cortisol levels and other reasons.

Some healthcare practitioners believe that patients who test within the normal range on thyroid tests are really severely hypothyroid. Besides the above-mentioned problems with thyroid lab tests, everyone's "normal" is different. What may be a high reading for one person may be a normal reading for another. For this reason, taking the body's morning temperature may be a more effective way of diagnosing hypothyroidism. A basal temperature of less than 98 degrees indicates hypothyroidism, while a temperature that fluctuates greatly throughout the day (and which is less than 98 degrees) indicates hypothyroidism caused by adrenal insufficiency.

Treating Hypothyroidism

Some people can manage symptoms of hypothyroidism by supplementing their diets with iodine and the amino acid L-tyrosine, constituents of thyroid hormone. The trace mineral selenium may also be needed to convert inactive thyroid hormone (T4) into the active form (T3). Other people may obtain good results by taking thyroid glandular formulas or homeopathic thyroid remedies. Because vitamin D and iron play a role in thyroid hormone utilization, taking these nutrients may also be helpful for those with deficiencies.

Many chronically ill people, however, aren't able to effectively synthesize thyroid hormones from amino acids and iodine. They require a prescription of bioidentical replacement T3/T4 hormones. Synthroid and other synthetic T4 products tend to be ineffective, since many people with Lyme disease cannot effectively convert T4 to T3 (the biologically active form of thyroid hormone), and instead make rT3 from T4. Such people do better by taking pure bioidentical T3 hormone until their adrenal insufficiency is adequately treated. Sadly, synthetic T4 is the only type of thyroid hormone replacement available in some countries, but compounded synthetic bioidentical T3/T4, or natural thyroid hormone preparations derived from porcine glands, are still available in the United States. These preparations are used in products such as Armour, Nature-throid, and Westhroid. Such products contain some T4, and may be less ideal for people with severely depleted adrenal glands, but they can be helpful for some. For others, pure bioidentical T3 (which can be obtained at compounding pharmacies throughout the United States) is a better option.

In Summary

Healing from adrenal insufficiency requires a comprehensive treatment approach that includes a healthy diet, adrenal supplements, a gentler approach to treating infections, appropriate thyroid support, and lifestyle modifications that address the initial causes of adrenal fatigue. (Lifestyle modifications will be discussed in greater detail in Chapter Eight). These treatments are just as important as addressing tick-borne infections. Treating adrenal fatigue and the hypothyroidism that often results from it should not be regarded as an ancillary, or adjunct, component of recovery.

Chapter Two

Nutrient Deficiencies and Toxic Food

Many people are sick today because they suffer from nutrient deficiencies and toxicity caused by an unhealthy diet, which causes them to be susceptible to Lyme and other diseases. Eating the wrong foods can cause illness, regardless of whether other factors are present to suppress the immune system. And it's not just about consuming fast-food or too many carbohydrates.

Our food supply isn't what it used to be. Foods contain fewer nutrients than they did just fifty years ago, and many of them have been genetically modified, manipulated, and biochemically altered into substances that hardly resemble food. They have also been exposed to and infused with toxins of all types, including pesticides, hormones, antibiotics, plastics, and other carcinogens that damage the body and make it susceptible to disease.

The current state of our food supply, and the effects that contaminated and unhealthy foods have upon the body have been described in documentaries such as *Food, Inc.* and in books by award-winning authors such as Michael Pollan and Jordan Rubin. Their research is backed by thousands of studies and by firsthand experience.

Food is medicine for the body. No vitamin supplement or herb can heal the body like food. Food is the fuel on which the body operates, regenerates, and repairs itself. No supplement can take the place of food, and no manipulating of food can make it better than how God, or nature, created it. It is naïve indeed to think that we can mess with the original design of food by altering its DNA and adding toxins to it that the body wasn't designed to process, without paying a price.

Because of what has been done to our food supply (the details of which will be described in the following sections), most people, whether chronically ill or not, have multiple nutrient deficiencies and a plethora of environmental toxins inside of them. Because chronic illness creates nutrient deficiencies, the sick suffer a double whammy: disease processes that create these deficiencies, along with a food supply that cannot restore to their bodies what they need in order to heal. A poor diet may even be, for some, the single most important contributing factor to disease. After all, if the body doesn't have the raw materials it needs to function, to make immune and other types of cells, or those cells can't function properly owing to nutrient deficiencies and toxic food, then infections and toxins will flourish within it. A healthy, clean body might effectively stave off Lyme disease, but when the immune system doesn't have the healthy-food ammunition that it needs to work properly, even a relatively benign infection can take it down.

I believe that many chronically ill people will struggle to recover if they consume non-organic, polluted, and adulterated food. Only organic food can provide the nutrients that the body needs to recover. Even then, most people will also need to take vitamin and mineral supplements, for reasons that will be explained in the following paragraphs.

Eating organic food used to be seen as something of a luxury or a fad, for those who could afford it and who wanted to stay super healthy. But it is imperative to understand that the only *real* food anymore *is* organic! If you don't eat organic, you aren't eating food the way it was created in nature, and in the form in which the body was designed to process it—you are eating a toxic product that has elements of nutrition in it, but which also harms the body in some way. Eating organic food is expensive, but so is being sick.

Fifty years ago, people who were chronically ill might have been able to get away with consuming food that wasn't labeled "organic," because the food supply was very different back then. Independent studies conducted in the United States, Canada, the United Kingdom, and other countries, have revealed that the nutritional content of our food has fallen substantially in recent decades. Results from studies published in *Food Magazine* (Jan.-March 2006), the *Journal of the American College of Nutrition* (Vol. 23:6, 2004) and *Life Extension Magazine* (March 2001), were presented at the May, 2011 conference, "A Deep Look Beyond Lyme." These results showed, for example, that three spears of broccoli in 1951 contained 130 mg of calcium, whereas in 1999 they contained only 48.3 mg. The Vitamin A content of broccoli in 1951 was 3,500 IU; in 1999 it was down to 1,542 IU. A potato in 1951 contained 17 mg of vitamin C; in 1999, it contained 7.25 mg. This represents a change of minus 57.35 percent! According to these studies, the nutrient content of other foods has also fallen substantially. Today, those numbers would be even lower.

This has happened in part because of modern industrial farming practices, which deplete the soil of nutrients that should end up in the food that's grown there. Soil is depleted of essential nutrients needed by the body to combat disease by extensive plowing, the use of chemical pesticides and fertilizers, and a failure to rotate crops and replace depleted soils with organic materials. Fruits and vegetables are also nutrient-deficient because they are picked prematurely and often shipped across thousands of miles. Meat and animal products are nutrient-deficient because farm animals are fed non-native diets and are forced to live in unnatural, confining, and toxic environments. In the following sections, I describe some of the dangers of industrial farming in greater detail.

Replenishing the body with the proper nutrients, which involves consuming healthy, organic foods, along with taking vitamin and mineral supplements, is essential for recovery from illness. While organic food and supplements are important for everyone nowadays, they are especially crucial for the chronically ill. Their nutrient needs are greater than those of the general population, and their tolerance and ability to remove toxins is lower. Jeffrey Morrison, MD, describes how the nutrient needs of the chronically ill differ from those of the general population in my book, *Insights into Lyme Disease Treatment*: ". . . Then there are the chronically ill, who require higher levels of nutrients in order to heal. This popular concept that people have similar nutritional needs is rubbish. Nobody would expect an Olympic athlete to have the same nutritional needs as someone who sits on the couch all day. And in the chronically ill, the immune system is running an Olympic marathon, and therefore, the bodies of such people require more nutrition than the bodies of those who aren't ill."

The Dangers of Genetically-Modified Food

Most industrially farmed foods that are sold in supermarkets have been genetically modified. Genetically modified organisms (GMOs) have been linked to a multitude of health problems and may either be a principal cause of symptoms, or a contributing factor to disease. Such is the concern among scientists about the dangers of GMOs that over 800 scientists from eighty-four countries have signed the "Open Letter from World Scientists to All Governments Concerning Genetically Modified Organisms." This letter, which was submitted to the UN, the World Trade Organization, and the U.S. Congress, calls for a ban on patenting life-forms and emphasizes the serious hazards of GMOs.

Many prominent U.S. Food and Drug Administration (FDA) scientists have also repeatedly expressed deep concerns about the dangerous effects of GMOs upon health. But their voices have been muted because the agricultural biotechnology industry (companies like Monsanto) have through lobbying efforts, downplayed the risks of GMOs to the government. Additionally, people with financial ties to biotech firms are employed in positions of authority at the FDA, which creates a conflict of interest between the biotech firms and that agency. The FDA is supposed to protect consumer health. This isn't possible when those in authority within the organization have a financial stake in the success of agricultural biotechnology companies, and thus, GMOs. Biotechnology and pharmaceutical company representatives influence the laws regarding our food supply, and their interests conflict with consumer health.

GMOs harm the body in many ways. First, they cause allergic reactions, some of them life-threatening. For example, in 1989, GMO L-tryptophan caused severe allergic reactions in thousands of people, and was removed from the market after dozens of people died from it. As another example, in March 1999, researchers at the York Nutritional Laboratory in Britain discovered that reactions to soy had skyrocketed by 50 percent over the previous year, and that these reactions corresponded with the introduction of genetically modified soy from the United States into Great Britain. Other studies have revealed similar adverse allergies and reactions.

But allergies are just the beginning of the story. GMOs also increase the severity of autoimmune disease. When foreign DNA (such as that which is found in GMO food) is introduced into the body, the body cannot digest it. Fragments of this undigested food instead pass through the intestinal wall into the bloodstream, where they cause inflammation and trigger autoimmune responses. Inflammation sets the stage for a variety of disease processes to occur, including cancer, and is the underlying precursor for most severe illnesses.

In 2001, Dr. Joe Cummins, Emeritus Professor of Genetics at the University of Western Ontario, made the following statement at the Toxicology Symposium at the University of Guelph: "The bacterial genes used in GM crops have been found to have significant impacts on the individuals ingesting GM crops. The impacts include inflammation, arthritis and lymphoma promotion." He also noted that because the body can't digest the foreign DNA that is introduced into GMOs, some of this DNA ends up in the chromosomes and adversely impacts the immune system. Unfortunately, it isn't scientists such as Dr. Cummins, who understand the implications of GMO food better than anyone, who are making the decisions about whether GMOs should be in our food supply.

At the time of the writing of this book, most true organic foods remain largely unaffected by GMOs, although this is slowly changing. My native state of Colorado has a chain of health food stores called Natural Grocers by Vitamin Cottage, which sells mostly 90–100 percent organic food that is free of GMOs and other contaminants. Shopping at supermarkets can be a challenge, because some position themselves as natural or health food markets, but much of what they sell, including their produce and meat isn't truly organic or GMO-free. For example, beef is sometimes advertised as being hormone-free, but if the cow from which it came wasn't grass-fed, its diet may have been comprised of GMO corn. So while the cow may be GMO-free, the food it ate was not, and the GM by-products of its unhealthy diet get transferred from its meat into our bodies. It's important to shop wisely and to read and understand labels when looking for GMO-free food.

How Conventionally Processed Meat Makes Us Sick

Another problem with the food supply is that corn and soy (most of which is genetically modified) are heavily subsidized by the government. They are found in a multitude of foods and food-like substances, due to their low cost. Joseph Mercola, MD, author of the world's most visited health site (www.mercola.com), writes in a 2011 article, "Why Are Toxin Proteins Genetically Engineered into Your Food?" He states: "The danger posed by GM crops is no longer theoretical, as proven by an analysis of 19 studies in which animals were fed GM soy and corn, which comprise more than 80 percent of all GMOs cultivated on a large scale, and exist in virtually every processed food sold in the United States."

In addition to corn and corn by-products being in so many boxed and canned foods, they are also found in the feed of livestock and farm-raised fish. They are fed corn because it's inexpensive. Cows and fish, however, weren't created to eat corn, which means that they get sick from it, and the quality of their meat becomes heavily degraded as a result of it. Studies show that cows, in particular, when fed a corn-based diet, develop enlarged livers and infections which must be treated with antibiotics. When we consume their meat, we also end up ingesting whatever they were fed, including those antibiotics. This removes beneficial flora from our bodies, and suppresses our immune systems.

Author Michael Pollan, in his 2001 *New York Times* article, "Power Steer" writes about cows that are fed unnatural grain diets: "Perhaps the most serious thing that can go wrong with a ruminant on corn is feedlot bloat. The rumen (one of the cow's stomach compartments where partially digested food is stored) is always producing copious amounts of gas, which is normally expelled by belching during rumination. But when the diet contains too much starch and too little roughage, rumination all but stops, and a layer of foamy slime that can trap gas forms in the rumen. The rumen inflates like a balloon, pressing against the animal's lungs. Unless action is promptly taken to relieve the pressure (usually by forcing a hose down the animal's esophagus), the cow suffocates."

He goes on to say, "A corn diet can also give a cow acidosis. Unlike that in our own highly acidic stomachs, the normal pH of a rumen is neutral. Corn makes it unnaturally acidic, however, causing a kind of bovine heart-burn, which in some cases can kill the animal but usually just makes it sick. Acidotic animals go off their feed, pant and salivate excessively, paw at their bellies and eat dirt. The condition can lead to diarrhea, ulcers, bloat, liver disease and a general weakening of the immune system that leaves the animal vulnerable to everything from pneumonia to feedlot polio."

Corn also alters cows' body tissues so that their meat becomes disproportionately high in omega-6 and saturated fatty acids. Most people have an excess of omega-6 fatty acids in their bodies as it is, which causes inflammation and is linked to a multitude of degenerative diseases, including cancer, autoimmune disease, and irritable bowel and metabolic syndromes. Meat from animals that are fed corn and other grains is estimated to contain only 15–50 percent of the amount of inflammation-lowering and health-promoting omega-3 fatty acids that are found in meat from grass-fed livestock. Grass-fed animals also have higher levels of Vitamin E and conjugated linoleic acid, both of which lower cancer risk.

But there's more. Since 1993, all non-organic milk products have contained high levels of IGF-1 (Insulin Growth Factor-1), a substance that stimulates cancer cell growth, after the FDA approved a genetically engineered bovine growth hormone (rBGH) to increase cows' milk production. Studies published in the *Journal of the National Cancer Institute* and *The Lancet* have since found that people who have higher circulating levels of IGF-1 in their bloodstream (from consuming non-organic milk) have much higher levels of breast and prostate cancer, both of which are particularly receptive to artificial hormones such as IGF-1. Evidence suggests that IGF-1 can also stimulate the development of other types of cancer.

Cows that are given growth hormone so that they can be processed faster and produce more meat/milk for human consumption are also forced to mature at an unnatural rate. This causes them to develop mastitis, or udder infections, for which they must be given antibiotics, which also eventually end up in our bodies.

People who have a predisposition to food allergies as a result of other immune stressors will react to this artificial and manipulated food with stronger symptoms than those who don't have obvious health problems. Yet even the healthiest of the healthy these days are prone to disease as a result of consuming nutrient-depleted, genetically modified, and contaminated food.

Just because a food tastes good and looks normal, doesn't mean that it is. Government campaigns sponsored by pharmaceutical companies have tried to convince people that giving cows and chickens antibiotics and hormones is perfectly safe and that GMOs cause no harm, but scientific studies and clinical evidence indicate otherwise.

The Problem with Additives, Preservatives, Pesticides, and Herbicides

Artificial additives and preservatives, which are added to all boxed and canned food products, are another source of toxicity for the body. Most people don't recognize their dangers. This is partly because their composition is cleverly disguised on food ingredient labels. For instance, MSG (monosodium glutamate), which many people now understand to be toxic and linked to neurological disorders, is often labeled as "textured protein," "soy protein isolate," and "natural flavoring." It seems as if food manufacturers know that most people will associate words like "natural flavoring" and "protein" with healthful substances. MSG and many other food additives and preservatives, such as sodium nitrate, BHA, BHT, potassium bromate, aspartame, food colorings, acesulfame-K, carrageenan, and others, are anything but natural to the body. Anything that isn't natural to the body causes disease-promoting inflammation.

It's also worth mentioning that the containers in which many foods are stored contain chemicals that are harmful to the body. Bisphenol-A (BPA), for example, a plastic and resin ingredient used to line metal food and drink cans, has been linked to birth defects, breast and prostate cancer, and infertility, among other conditions. Whenever possible, avoid canned food and plastic beverage bottles. Frozen foods that are bagged in plastic also contain small amounts of plastic residue as a result of the bags. Consuming fresh food, whenever possible, is best.

The less a natural food resembles its original form—the more it has been processed and the more additives it contains—the more inflammation it causes. Oats, for example, may be a non-inflammatory food for a person who isn't allergic to grains, but when extensively processed and combined with many additives to make a granola bar, it ceases to be healthful.

Pesticides and herbicides are sprayed on produce, contained within GMO organisms, and found in the feed of conventionally-raised livestock. These substances are another source of disease-promoting inflammation. Among their many detrimental effects upon the body, they create perforations in the gut and cause Leaky Gut Syndrome, a condition whereby whole food particles pass through the villi of the intestinal lining into the bloodstream (instead of being digested by the body), which causes inflammation.

Pesticides have also been directly associated with the development of certain cancers, such as soft-tissue sarcomas, non-Hodgkin's lymphoma, leukemia, and cancers of the lung and breast. Ingesting pesticides may cause other damaging effects in the body that scientists are yet unaware of. For instance, one pesticide called Bt, which is placed in GMO foods by biotech companies, is thousands of times more concentrated than natural bug spray, but scientists have yet to test its effects upon the human body.

Making Healthy Food Choices

These days, it can be difficult to identify truly healthy foods. After I became ill, it took me several years of research before I understood which foods were good for the body, and which weren't. Having been raised, as much of society, on boxed and canned foods, and unaware of the dangers of GMOs, I realized that the food industry has cleverly manipulated and marketed its products so as to confuse even the health-conscious. Words like "low-calorie," "low-fat," and "all natural ingredients" can deceive, especially when we have been taught that these things are good for us. And most intelligent people assume that "all natural" means what it says: the way nature created it! But sadly, product labels don't always mean what they say, or say what they mean.

Yes, it's obvious that vegetables are good for you, but what about seemingly natural food products that have more than a few ingredients on their labels, or that don't look the same as when they came out of the ground? What about granola bars, soy and almond milk, mozzarella cheese, turkey sausage, and so-called "natural" yogurt? These foods may not be as good for you as you think, if they have been adulterated, for example, through pasteurization (which destroys beneficial enzymes needed to digest dairy products), the addition of preservatives (such as carrageenan in nondairy milk), or too many other ingredients. These ingredients harm the body because that's not how the food is ordinarily found in nature. Thus, choosing foods that are in as natural a state as possible is the best rule of thumb to follow when deciding upon what to eat.

It's also important to consider where the food came from. Organic food is unquestionably healthier for the body, but true organic food can be challenging to find. This is because real organic food is produced according to traditional farming methods, which involve crop rotation, producing multiple crops together, using manure instead of chemicals for fertilizer, using soil in an ecologically sustainable manner, and so forth. Today, large organic farms employ many of the same practices as non-organic, industrialized farms, such as monoculture (single-crop production over a large area) and shipping food across thousands of miles. This is due to massive production demands by large chain supermarkets such as Whole Foods. Sadly, the so-called "free range" animals from such farms may have little more than a small yard outside in which they can walk for a few hours during the day. The animals still spend most of their time in cages or pens. Due to large-scale production demands and the fact that most consumers purchase their food from supermarkets (rather than directly from farms, co-ops, or farmers' markets), large organic farms have been forced to resort to some of the same practices as non-organic farms. These practices go against the basic principles of true organic farming. The food may not have pesticides, herbicides, or antibiotics, but it may be of inferior nutritional value compared to food that is produced according to true organic farming methods.

Shopping at organic farmers' markets or purchasing food directly from organic local farms is the best way to obtain fresh, nutrient-rich food, and to support true organic farming practices rather than large-scale industrialized farming.

Buying from local farmers has many benefits. Their fruits and vegetables are likely to have a higher nutritional content because they aren't picked prior to maturity and shipped thousands of miles, and they are grown in superior, mineral-rich soil. Their livestock tend to be raised under more humane conditions than animals on large, industrialized farms. Buying from local farmers also discourages waste, saves on fuel costs and energy (since the food doesn't have to travel a long distance), and benefits the environment and humanity in other ways. For more information on the differences between large-scale, industrialized organic farming and true organic farming, and the advantages of purchasing food from a local organic farm or farmer's market instead of the supermarket, I highly recommend reading Michael Pollan's book, *The Omnivore's Dilemma*.

Follow Michael Pollan's "Food Rules"

The *New York Times* award-winning journalist Michael Pollan has written some excellent books about how foods are produced, distributed, and consumed in America. His pocket-sized book *Food Rules* is another excellent resource on healthy eating. It describes in simple, yet profound terms how to eat well without having to follow a complex dietary protocol. The basic premise of the book is to eat real food; vegetables, fruits, whole grains, fish, and meat, and to avoid what he calls "edible food-like substances."

This book, which contains sixty-four short rules for eating well, provides tidbits of common sense, yet valuable information that can help people with health challenges to make wise food choices. For example, Pollan advocates not eating anything that your great-grandmother wouldn't recognize as food, because our ancestors had no choice but to consume natural food! He also suggests not eating anything that contains more than five ingredients, or ingredients that you can't pronounce. He encourages shopping around the perimeter of the supermarket, since real food (e.g., produce and fresh animal protein) tends to be found there. His fresh, uncomplicated suggestions help even the most brain-fogged of souls to understand how to eat well. That said, people with Lyme and other chronic illnesses may benefit from additional guidelines, which I outline in the following section.

As a reassurance to those with health problems, I believe that the prevalence of food allergies in people with chronic health challenges is due more to problems that are inherent in the food supply than to problems with their immune systems. So don't feel bad if you are allergic to dairy! The so-called healthy population is allergic, also—they just don't realize it, because their symptoms may not be as obvious as yours, and/or their overall body burden of toxins may not yet be high enough to cause symptoms.

For example, have you noticed how the entire world seems to be allergic to gluten these days, and how an increasing number of restaurants are advertising gluten-free food? It's not just because the rate of chronic illness is skyrocketing—it's because bread contains more gluten now than it used to (thanks to the efforts of biotechnology companies), and many other foods now also contain it. Gluten is a protein found mostly in wheat, but it's also present in grains such as rye and barley. Grains that are supposed to be gluten-free, such as oats, sometimes contain traces of gluten if they are processed in the same factories as gluten-containing grains. The average body can't digest massive amounts of gluten. Whatever isn't digested passes through the villi of the intestinal wall into the bloodstream, and causes inflammation.

Half of the foods that the chronically ill can't consume because of allergies, healthier people shouldn't be consuming, either. In a way, having symptoms can be a blessing in disguise, because they can alert you to the foods that aren't truly good for any human being, a reality that a so-called healthier person might miss.

Dietary Recommendations for People with Lyme Disease

Many people with Lyme and chronic illness may require more specific dietary guidelines than the aforementioned. Not all healthy foods are easy for people with these conditions to digest. Raw vegetables, for instance, can be challenging, because many people with Lyme have hydrochloric acid deficiencies in the stomach and a lack of enzymes in the small intestine. Also, raw foods require a lot of energy to digest, and the chronically ill don't have an abundance of energy. When I was really sick with Lyme disease, it would sometimes take me 45 minutes to eat a salad, due to these factors. Taking hydrochloric acid in capsule form never helped me much, but it may be beneficial for some people.

Soft, squishy foods such as dairy products and grains, which may seem easier for the stomach to process, usually cause inflammation or contain ingredients such as gluten that the body can't break down. They should therefore be avoided. Some people are able to eat non-gluten grains, such as oats or rice bread, but I have observed that most people with severe chronic health conditions do best if they avoid all grains completely. Jordan Rubin, the bestselling author of *The Maker's Diet,* who completely recovered from Crohn's disease by changing his diet, advocates a grain-free diet for those with severe chronic illness.

It can be frustrating to find foods to eat during recovery. Nutrition books admonish people who are chronically ill to consume plenty of fresh, raw green vegetables—but who wants to eat vegetables two or three times a day, when you can barely get them into your stomach, never mind through the intestines?

Taking digestive enzymes and a hydrochloric acid supplement may help the body to process difficult foods. It's also helpful to find foods that are easy, and enjoyable, for the body to digest. Juicing vegetables and low-glycemic fruits may be a beneficial option for some people. Veggies and fruits are more readily absorbed by the body in liquid form. The only drawback to juicing is that it removes the fiber that is found in fruits and vegetables. It can also cause a blood sugar spike, due to the nutrients being more quickly absorbed into the bloodstream. Eating some animal protein or nuts before drinking the juice may prevent this from happening.

Consuming cooked vegetables in a stew or soup is another option. Cooked veggies tend to be easier to digest than raw veggies. This is also true for meat that is prepared as a stew in a slow cooker, rather than grilled, fried, broiled or even baked in an oven. One advantage of stews is that several portions can be prepared in a Crock-Pot or other slow cooker and reheated multiple times, as leftovers. This is beneficial for those who are too tired to cook on a daily basis.

Cooked veggies don't have the same nutritional value as raw ones, but if you aren't properly digesting the raw ones anyway, consuming cooked veggies may be better, since they don't require as much energy to digest. That said, most nutritionists believe that consuming at least some raw vegetables is important because of their higher nutrient content. For people who are chronically ill, a better strategy might be combining a diet of raw juiced vegetables and the occasional salad, with an abundance of cooked vegetables.

Some Lyme-literate doctors believe that healthy, non-gluten grains are acceptable foods for those with tick-borne illnesses. That said, I have yet to meet a severely chronically ill person with Lyme who can tolerate little more than brown rice or an occasional piece of bread as part of their regular diet. Other Lyme-literate doctors believe that grains (and carbohydrates in general) feed pathogens in the body and promote inflammation, and should therefore be completely avoided.

When consumed in moderation, some healthier people may tolerate grains.

Discerning Food Allergies

Although I am no longer treating my body for tick-borne infections, I have found that I can yet only consume brown rice several times per week, and other grains only occasionally (once or twice per week), without getting tired. Fatigue after eating is a sign that the body was sensitive or allergic to something that was eaten, although not everyone recognizes it as such. You aren't supposed to be fatigued after you eat. If you are, it's generally because: 1) you just ate something that you were sensitive or allergic to, 2) you ate too much, or 3) your adrenals are exhausted and you don't have enough energy to metabolize large meals.

Sometimes symptoms that result from food allergies and sensitivities have a delayed onset. They may not appear until a day or two after the food was eaten. The inflammatory immune response that is caused by the allergy may also last for days, even weeks, after exposure to the offending food. When determining food allergies, it's a good idea to eliminate all foods that you suspect to be allergenic from your diet. Avoid consuming them for an extended period of time (perhaps a month or two). Then, you can slowly introduce them back into your diet, one by one, and discern specifically which ones are causing problems, based on your reaction to each.

The Coca pulse test is another simple way to check for food allergies. To do this, check your pulse rate at rest five minutes prior to eating a meal and then again fifteen minutes following the completion of that meal. Rest following the meal, so that your pulse isn't elevated by activity. If your pulse rate is at least 15 beats per minute faster after the meal, it is likely that you ate a food that you are allergic to. If your pulse rate is 10-1 beats per minute faster after the meal, you may have eaten a food that you are allergic to. If your pulse rate increases less than 10 beats per minute, it is unlikely that you ate any allergenic foods.

Foods That Most Everyone Can Eat

So if you have severe chronic illness and/or tick-borne infections, what can you eat?

An appropriate diet for recovery depends somewhat on individual bio-chemistry, as well as the degree and causes of illness; however, in general, the following foods are safe, healthy choices for most everyone with chronic illness involving Lyme disease:

1. Organic, grass-fed, non-GMO, antibiotic- and hormone-free, free-range meat products of all types. This includes beef, chicken, wild game such as elk and buffalo, lamb, and turkey. Pork should be consumed only occasionally, as it is thought to not be a "clean" meat (pigs eat most everything, even dead animals, and their meat often contains parasites). Some people can also tolerate eggs.

2. Fish that contain low levels of mercury, such as wild-caught sockeye salmon and sardines. Tuna may be eaten in moderation, if it has been tested for mercury. Avoid most other types of fish, as they tend to

contain high levels of mercury. As a rule of thumb, the larger the fish, the more toxic heavy metals it contains.

3. Low-glycemic-index fruits, such as avocado, berries, grapefruit, and lemon. These can be consumed in abundance. Fruits with moderate levels of sugar, or higher glycemic indexes, such as apples and pears, should be limited to one serving per day. Most fruit juice and high-glycemic fruits should be avoided, since these cause blood sugar spikes that tend to lead to hypoglycemia, inflammation, and insulin resistance. If high-glycemic fruits such as bananas, papayas, grapes, and melons are eaten, they should only be consumed after a meal containing protein, which blunts the blood sugar spike that they produce.

4. Nuts and seeds (except for peanuts, which tend to encourage mold growth). Walnuts, almonds, Brazil nuts, pine nuts, and pecans; flaxseed and sunflower, pumpkin, and sesame seeds are all good choices, along with nut butters that don't contain sugar. A few people may have allergies to all kinds of nuts). In any case, be mindful of not consuming nuts in excess, as most contain high levels of omega-6 fatty acids. An imbalance of omega-3 and omega-6 fatty acids in the body causes inflammation. Two small handfuls daily of most types of nuts are probably sufficient.

5. Non-gluten grains. These include foods such as quinoa, amaranth, millet, and brown rice. Quinoa isn't a true grain, but a seed that contains higher levels of protein than any other grain or seed. A small percentage of people may tolerate one or two servings of non-gluten grains daily, especially quinoa. Other people may tolerate non-gluten grains only occasionally, while others, not at all. Brown rice should be eaten in conjunction with animal protein, to avoid blood sugar spikes.

6. Legumes, such as black beans, black-eyed peas, lentils, and chickpeas. Again, a few people may tolerate consuming these on a daily basis, and if so, they should be limited to one serving per day. Others may tolerate them on occasion, while others, not at all.

7. Vegetables of all types, including moderate amounts of starchy vegetables such as squash and sweet potato. Some people with Lyme

should also avoid nightshade vegetables, such as eggplant, peppers, white potatoes and tomatoes, because they can exacerbate inflammation. Excellent juices can be made from carrots and beets, but I recommend consuming such juices in combination with a protein-rich food. Drinking the juice on an empty stomach can cause blood sugar spikes, which wears out the adrenal glands and encourages the development of hypoglycemia, diabetes, and insulin resistance. Vegetables that are healthy to eat and which can be consumed in abundance include:

- Artichoke
- Arugula
- Beets
- Bok choy
- Broccoli
- Brussels sprouts
- Cabbage
- Carrots
- Celery
- Collard greens
- Cucumbers
- Garlic
- Kale
- Leeks
- Lettuce
- Mustard greens
- Onions
- Scallions
- Spinach
- Sprouts
- String beans
- Watercress

8. Healthy oils and fats, such as coconut and olive oil, ghee (clarified butter), and organic butter.

9. Some condiments and sweeteners, including spices of all kinds: sea salt, vanilla extract, stevia, and xylitol. Avoid honey and agave

nectar, as both spike blood sugar levels. Artificial sweeteners should also be avoided.

Foods to Avoid

Soy, in general, should be avoided. Most soy is genetically modified and is found in a multitude of packaged and processed food products, which means that most people get too much of it. Soy also tends to depress thyroid function and contains plant estrogens that mimic the effects of human estrogen upon the body. Most people in our society have an excess of estrogen, due to the xenoestrogenic effects that chemical contaminants in the environment have upon the body. Consuming foods that increase estrogen may not be a good idea. In fact, studies have shown that men who consume high amounts of soy have lowered testosterone levels and decreased sperm counts. The estrogenic effects of soy may even contribute to male breast formation. When eaten in moderation, however, and consumed in healthy fermented foods such as miso, natto and tempeh, soy can be beneficial.

Dairy products should also mostly be avoided. Most people are allergic to dairy (even goat dairy) because the pasteurization process that commercial dairy products are required to undergo in the United States removes vital enzymes the body needs to effectively digest them. Some people may be able to tolerate dairy products that come from goats, since they tend to be easier for the body to digest than cow dairy products. Others cannot consume any pasteurized products. Many states have raw and organic dairy farms that sell products directly to the consumer, although the government is starting to shut down some of these farms. If you can obtain your dairy products from a farmer who produces raw dairy, you may find that you are able to tolerate these products better. Raw, unpasteurized dairy products produced under sanitary conditions are a healthy and wonderful source of protein when they come from animals that haven't been fed an unhealthy diet, hormones, or antibiotics.

In general, most people with Lyme disease or severe chronic illness can't tolerate milk, whether from cows, sheep, or goats. Conventionally-produced milk is extremely toxic to the body, not only because it's pasteurized, but also because it contains hormones and antibiotics, along with infections and infectious by-products that result from the livestock living under unnatural conditions and being fed a non-native diet. It is a myth that commercial milk products provide calcium to the body. The United States has one of the highest rates of consumption of milk, worldwide, and yet also has one of the highest rates of osteoporosis.

Some people may tolerate moderate amounts of mozzarella, feta, and other types of cheese made from goat's and sheep's milk that don't contain high amounts of additives and preservatives. I have found one type of healthy goat's milk cheese at a local health food store, Natural Grocers by Vitamin Cottage, which contains only sea salt and enzymes, in addition to the cheese itself. It hasn't been extensively processed, and I feel good after I eat it.

Beyond small to moderate amounts of goat's milk cheese, some people may be able to tolerate organic goat or sheep's milk yogurt and kefir. Others will have to stick to non-dairy sources of yogurt and kefir, such as coconut. These should also not contain any unnecessary additives. Food manufacturers are currently using a seaweed derivative called carrageenan to thicken and emulsify some types of coconut yogurt, but studies have shown this additive to cause gastrointestinal problems. It has also been linked to the development of cancers of the digestive tract. Any type of yogurt that has artificial additives and preservatives, or sugar (even if it's cane or fruit juice sugar) should be avoided.

Because most people with Lyme disease and environmental illness suffer from gut problems—irritable bowel syndrome, leaky gut, and the like—consuming foods that contain probiotics is absolutely essential for healing the gut. Dairy sources of yogurt and kefir may contain healthful bacteria that help to ward off pathogenic bacteria and replenish deficient levels of beneficial flora in the digestive tract, but they also tend to inflame the body because they are pasteurized. Other food sources of probiotics, such as kombucha, homemade kefir made from coconut milk and bacterial cultures, kimchi, and sauerkraut, may be better choices for replenishing gut flora. For more information about probiotics, see Chapter Seven.

People with chronic health challenges should not consume refined sugar, caffeine, and alcohol on a regular basis. All of these substances cause inflammation and stress the adrenal glands. It can be extremely difficult for some people to quit these substances, because chronic illness creates neurotransmitter and hormone deficiencies, in addition to faulty carbohydrate metabolism. It is not uncommon for people to strongly crave substances that will meet their bodies' immediate need for glucose and happiness-inducing biochemicals, when there is an absence of adequate glucose to the cells, along with low levels of cortisol and serotonin, and an excess of molds and yeast in the body (which tend to be prevalent in those with Lyme disease). Refined sugar and caffeine, especially, meet this need. Attempting to give up these substances without addressing the underlying biochemical problems that are causing the cravings can be incredibly difficult. Sugar and caffeine dependence are addictions that can be just as fierce and difficult to quit as smoking, alcohol, and recreational drugs.

Supporting the adrenal glands with nutrients and rest, getting rid of yeast and other fungal infections, and taking a combination of amino acids may, over time, enable the sugar or caffeine addict to wean off of these harmful substances. In the meantime, limiting their use and finding acceptable substitutes, however possible, is important for healing.

Over the past eight years, I have maintained a mostly healthy diet and practiced what I have preached, but it has been difficult for me to completely quit drinking caffeinated coffee, since my cortisol and serotonin levels have typically been low. Caffeine raises both cortisol and serotonin levels in the body. It has taken me a long time to learn how to figure out how to raise them. I am a disciplined person who has always desired to be well, but my body's intense need for certain biochemicals has made it a challenge for me to wean myself off of coffee.

If you can relate to my experience, some strategies that have helped me to say "No" to caffeine, sugar, and alcohol include:

1.   Making sure that I eat small portions of animal protein and fat every 3-4 hours. This helps me to stave off cravings while meeting my body's need for amino acids, from which hormones and neurotransmitters are made.

2.   Drinking half-and-half coffee—that is, half caffeinated, half decaf—or

a favorite tea that contains less caffeine than coffee, such as green tea.

3. Replacing chocolate and other desserts with an occasional 85 percent dark chocolate bar, which contains only 4 grams of sugar per serving. These can be found at your local health food store, and are a nice treat to have on occasion when you just can't say "No" to chocolate. Also, you can make chocolate at home using unsweetened chocolate, stevia liquid and homemade nut milk.

4. Indulging in an unhealthy meal every once in awhile. I do this so that I don't feel as though I can never have my favorite foods (which are mostly unhealthy!) and give up on my healthy diet. I used to feel guilty whenever I would go out with friends on the weekends and have a beer or chocolate dessert. But I would also feel deprived and sad if I watched them indulge in these foods and I couldn't join in on the fun. My favorite foods soon became just one more thing that chronic illness stole from me. To avoid this depressing thought, I began to allow myself to indulge in an unhealthy meal every once in awhile. I did this because I reasoned that depression is also unhealthy and suppresses immune function, just as sugar does. It was in my best interest to avoid getting depressed over my diet. If not being able to eat your favorite foods (because they happen to be unhealthy) depresses you, you may want to have them every so often. It isn't prudent to eat desserts and other junk food on a regular basis, though. Around Christmas and during the holidays, when the temptation to eat junk food is high, you may want to consider bringing your own sugarless or gluten-free desserts to events, or eating before parties so that you won't be tempted to eat as much harmful food while you are there. One simple, yet healthy and delicious dessert I invented involves melting butter, cinnamon, and stevia over pecans, and then roasting the ingredients in the oven for a few minutes. Stevia and Xylitol are excellent natural sugar substitutes for many desserts, and for sweetening beverages.

5. Look for cookbooks that have creative dessert recipes for people who can't tolerate dairy, gluten, or sugar. *The Detoxx Book* patients'

manual from the home detoxification program of John S. Foster, MD and Patricia Kane, PhD, while not a cookbook per se, has healthy dessert recipes for people who have food allergies of all kinds. All of the recipes listed in this manual are tolerated by most people with Lyme disease. They will help the body detoxify. For instance, one cookie recipe uses a high-quality egg protein powder in lieu of flour. When people can't tolerate even non-gluten grains, high-quality egg protein, hemp seed, quinoa, amaranth and almond flours are great flour substitutes for cookies and cakes.

6. Consulting health-oriented cookbooks can also help people with health challenges to feel as though they have options. When you know that you can't eat much of what is sold in the supermarket, it's easy to feel as though you don't have many dietary choices. Authors of cookbooks for the health-conscious often provide creative suggestions that can help you to think outside the box for meal ideas when food options seem limited. Another book I recommend, *The Paleo Diet Cookbook* by Loren Cordain, PhD, has many ideal recipes for the chronically ill. It's based upon a diet that most people with Lyme and chronic illness can tolerate, such as lean animal protein and non-starchy fruits and veggies.

It can be challenging to maintain a strict diet that excludes most grains, dairy products, fruit, and sugar. It can be disheartening to feel as though you can seldom eat your favorite foods. The reality is, however, that recovery from chronic illness is difficult unless the body is sustained by anti-inflammatory food on a regular basis.

Before the advent of industrialized farming and the addition of chemicals, GMOs, additives, antibiotics, hormones, and the like to our food supply, dairy products were safe. Grains and soy were good for you. Today, much of what is sold in the supermarket isn't safe—for anyone! It isn't just that people with health challenges have special dietary needs; rather, their bodies simply respond with a greater shout to the foods that none of us should be consuming. The symptoms that they experience serve as a barometer for what the rest of society probably should or should not be eating.

Having health challenges can be a blessing, if symptoms teach us to eat in the way that nature intended. As the world is now, we are slowly poisoning ourselves to death by defying nature and manipulating the food supply and our environment.

The Most Common Nutrient Deficiencies and How to Reverse Them

Nutrient deficiencies in people with Lyme disease and chronic illness are usually severe enough to necessitate having to take vitamin and mineral supplements, in addition to maintaining a healthy, organic diet, in order to get well. The following are common deficiencies in such people:

Magnesium

Tick-borne organisms deplete this mineral from the body, so most people with Lyme have moderate to severe magnesium deficiencies. Magnesium is responsible for a multitude of functions in the body. It plays a role in over 300 enzymatic processes and is involved in energy production and transport, muscle contraction and relaxation, protein production, hormone regulation, and nerve conduction. It also plays an essential role in the maintenance and repair of all body cells.

Symptoms of magnesium deficiency include: tremors, twitches, cramps, muscle soreness, heart palpitations, depression, insomnia, irritability, apathy, fatigue, confusion, poor memory, and weakness. Many other symptoms can result, as well. Taking a high-quality magnesium supplement can reduce the severity of, or eliminate, these symptoms. Because magnesium absorption can be compromised by bowel problems, such as a leaky gut, and because deficiencies in people with Lyme can be severe, some physicians recommend magnesium injections, transdermal magnesium creams, or intravenous infusions of magnesium, rather than oral forms of the mineral. Also, not all forms of oral magnesium are equally effective. Magnesium malate or citrate is often recommended by holistic doctors. Ginger Savely, DNP, who has treated thousands of chronically ill Lyme patients, recommends Peter Gilham's Natural Calm products. Necessary dosages may range from 350–1,000 mg daily, and should be taken in divided doses throughout the day.

Omega-3 Essential Fatty Acids (EFAs)

Tick-borne infections destroy neural tissue and cause lesions on the brain. Omega-3 EFAs help to reverse this damage. Omega-3 EFAs can also improve symptoms of brain fog, memory loss, and depression, which are common in chronic illness. Omega-3 EFAs also prevent some risk factors for heart disease and lower inflammation, which is a persistent problem in chronic illness.

Symptoms of omega-3 fatty acid deficiency, in addition to the above-mentioned, include: irritability, insomnia, confusion, muscle twitches, and rapid heartbeat. While it's important to supplement for omega-3 deficiencies, it's also important to ensure that the ratio of omega-3 to omega-6 fatty acids is balanced in the body. Most people today, sick or not, have too many omega-6 fatty acids in their diets, compared to omega-3 fatty acids. According to endocrinologist Diana Schwarzbein, MD, in her book, *The Schwarzbein Principle II*, having too many omega-6 EFAs in the body can promote inflammation and also cause hypercoagulation. This condition causes the blood to become too thick, preventing nutrients, oxygen, and antimicrobial treatments from reaching the cells.

New Zealand nutritionist Julianne Taylor notes on her website, *Julianne's Paleo & Zone Nutrition* (paleozonenutrition.com), that the body needs both omega-6 EFAs and omega-3 EFAs, in a ratio of about 4:1 (omega-6 to omega-3). She states that people who follow the Standard American Diet (SAD), have a ratio of about 20:1; that is, 20 times more omega-6 fatty acids than omega-3s. A chart on Taylor's website lists the amounts of omega-3 and -6 fatty acids found in different foods.

Consuming foods that are rich in omega-3 EFAs can help balance the omega-6 to omega-3 ratio, but reducing omega-6 EFA consumption is likewise important, since most people get too many of these pro-inflammatory fatty acids in their diets. Sources of omega-6 fatty acids are numerous. They are found in seeds, nuts and their oils, as well as in refined vegetable oils (especially soy), which are used in most processed and fast foods. Removing unhealthy sources of omega-6 EFAs, especially those found in fast food, is important for recovery.

Wild-caught salmon and sardines are probably the best animal-protein sources of omega-3 fatty acids. Other animal products, such as free-range chicken and eggs, and grass-fed beef, also contain some omega-3 EFAs. As with other nutrients, the body more readily utilizes and absorbs omega-3 EFAs from food sources than from supplements. Even so, taking a quality fish oil product may be a necessary dietary adjunct, since it is difficult to get enough omega-3 EFAs from food alone. Unfortunately no fish oil product is completely free of toxins. Most have traces of mercury and other contaminants in them. Purchasing a brand that has been molecularly distilled to remove most contaminants, especially heavy metals, is important. Nordic Naturals is one brand that I have used for years, which has a reputation for being relatively pure.

Vitamin D-3

Most people in the United States, not just the chronically ill, are deficient in vitamin D-3. This vitamin acts more like a hormone in the body than a vitamin. It is important for supporting endocrine health, and especially the adrenal and thyroid glands. Studies have also shown it to play an important role in immune system function. Low levels of vitamin D-3 have been associated with high levels of inflammation in the body. Therefore, supplementing with an oral form of vitamin D-3, along with sunlight, may be important for healing. Dosage recommendations usually range from 2,000–20,000 IU daily, depending upon the level of deficiency that is present. It is important to have your vitamin D-3 levels tested in order to determine how much supplementation you need. The testing method for vitamin D used by some labs isn't very reliable, so it's important to choose a reputable lab. Lyme-literate doctor Lee Cowden, MD recommends Lab Corp for vitamin D testing.

Vitamin C

Vitamin C may be the most significant vitamin for immune system health. The adrenal glands and brain utilize most of the body's vitamin C. In people who are chronically ill, the body's need for vitamin C can be incredibly high. Linus Pauling, a two-time Nobel Prize laureate, believed that people should take 10–20 grams (or 10,000–20,000 mg) of vitamin C daily, just to maintain health! His recommendations for people with health challenges, then, were much higher. According to Pauling, Vitamin C's ability to prevent illness arises from its role in manufacturing collagen, the protein that gives shape to connective tissues and strength to skin and blood vessels. Since tick-borne infections destroy connective tissue, people with Lyme disease may benefit from high doses of vitamin C, although some Lyme-literate doctors recommend moderately high doses instead; perhaps 2 - 4 grams daily. Still others recommend taking vitamin C to bowel tolerance.

In addition to its role in manufacturing collagen, vitamin C is important for maintaining proper immune function and pH, and for detoxifying and repairing the body. Vitamin C promotes cellular repair, supports healthy gut bacteria production, destroys harmful bacteria and viruses; removes heavy metals and other environmental contaminants. As an antioxidant, it neutralizes free radicals that result from inflammation. Thus, it plays an immensely important role in healing the body from toxicity and chronic illness.

When choosing a vitamin C product, it's best to avoid GMO corn-derived vitamin C (which is the most common type of vitamin C in the United States), and to assess the bioavailability of different forms of vitamin C. For instance, ascorbyl palmitate is thought by some sources to be more effective in the body than ascorbic acid. One vitamin C product I have used over the past two years, and which has provided a noticeable increase in my energy, is Pure Horizon's LipoNano C. Some studies have revealed liposomal products (encased in lipids for improved absorption) to be more effective than typical water-soluble vitamin C products. Liposomal supplements are more expensive; people who can't afford them may want to learn how to make them from regular supplements. A relatively simple procedure for doing this is explained in-depth, on wellness advocate Scott Forsgren's blog at: http://www.betterhealthguy.com/joomla/blog/232-making-a-liposomal-compound.

Iron

Many people with Lyme and chronic illness, especially women, are deficient in iron. Eliminating *Babesia*, one of the co-infections implicated in chronic Lyme disease, can help to raise iron levels, since *Babesia* depletes the body of this mineral. While it's also important to supplement for iron deficiencies, it can be difficult to raise the body's iron levels with synthetic iron supplements, and even iron injections, because the mineral is notoriously difficult for the body to absorb when it's not contained within food. Some doctors believe that synthetic iron supplements feed pathogenic organisms anyway, and that it is better to take food-based iron products, which are made from whole foods. Food-based iron supplements may also be more readily absorbed by the body. My compounding pharmacist recommends New Chapter's Every Woman's Iron Support supplement, and claims that this food-based iron supplement has effectively raised many of his client's iron levels when iron injections failed to do so. Floradix is another reputable iron product, which is made from iron gluconate, a highly absorbable form of iron.

It's important to measure iron levels before giving the body supplemental iron. A few people with Lyme have too much iron in their bodies, which is just as harmful as not having enough.

Other Minerals

Many of our foods are also mineral-deficient because most of the soil that our food is grown in is severely depleted of minerals. Minerals are responsible for a multitude of chemical processes in the body, including metabolizing nutrients and producing energy, building tissues and hormones, facilitating enzymatic processes, synthesizing hemoglobin, and supporting the immune system. People with Lyme disease tend to have severe mineral deficiencies of any and/or all of the following: magnesium, calcium, iodine, chromium, selenium, manganese, boron, biotin, zinc, lithium, and molybdenum. People with pyroluria (which is explained in greater detail in Chapter Five), have deficiencies of all of the above, with the possible exception of iodine. Pyroluria is present in 80 percent of those with chronic Lyme disease and 50 percent of those with depression who don't have Lyme disease. Correcting mineral deficiencies is imperative for healing the body. BioPure™ makes a product called CORE, which contains all of the trace minerals that people with pyroluria need to replenish what is missing from their bodies. For more information on the CORE product, visit www.biopureus.com.

B-Vitamins

People with Lyme disease and chronic illness are often deficient in B vitamins, especially vitamins B-6, B-5 and B-12. The B vitamins are heavily involved in the body's stress response, and are quickly depleted in chronic disease states.

Vitamin B-5, or pantothenic acid, is necessary for protein, fat, and carbohydrate synthesis and metabolism. It also plays an important role in adrenal gland function. Symptoms of vitamin B-5 deficiency may include: fatigue, headaches, nausea, tingling in the hands, depression, and cardiac problems. Frequent infection, fatigue, abdominal pains, sleep disturbances, and neurological disorders including numbness, paresthesia (sensations of burning, tingling, pricking, and numbness), muscle weakness, and cramps are other indications that this nutrient may be lacking in the body. Taking pantothenic acid may therefore be a good idea for anyone with adrenal fatigue and Lyme disease.

Vitamin B-6 is involved in many aspects of nutrient metabolism, as well as neurotransmitter synthesis, hemoglobin function and synthesis, and gene expression. It also plays a vital role in lipid metabolism and gluconeogenesis (the process by which glucose is made from non-carbohydrate sources of food). Symptoms of vitamin B-6 deficiency are non-specific. This deficiency isn't thought to be common among the general population, since B-6 is found in many foods. In people with adrenal fatigue and pyroluria, however, deficiencies are common. Pyridoxal phosphate, or P-5-P, tends to be the easiest form of B-6 for the body to metabolize, and may be the best form to take when supplementing for deficiencies.

For information on vitamin B-12, including symptoms of deficiency and how to replenish B-12 stores, see the section on vitamin B-12 in Chapter Eight.

Gut Flora

Many people have a deficiency of beneficial flora (bacteria) in the gut, due to an overgrowth of pathogens, which take advantage of a weak immune system and occupy the intestines. People with Lyme disease who have been on extended courses of antibiotics are particularly likely to have a deficiency of healthy flora and an imbalance of intestinal microorganisms. Antibiotics wipe out not only tick-borne pathogens, but also beneficial bacteria living in the gut and on the skin. For quality probiotic recommendations, and more information on how to restore the health of the GI tract, see Chapter Seven.

Drink Clean Water

Finally, just as it is important to consume natural, organic, clean food, it is also essential to drink clean water. Unfortunately, all tap water nowadays is contaminated by fluoride, chlorine, asbestos, plastics, pesticides, antibiotics, pharmaceutical drugs, heavy metals and other industrial contaminants, as well as parasites, bacteria, and other harmful microorganisms. For this reason, it is essential to use a reverse osmosis or carbon block water filter to filter all drinking and bathing water, to avoid bodily contamination by these pollutants. If you can't afford a good water filter, some health food stores sell water that has been purified via reverse osmosis. This water can be purchased by the gallon or in larger quantities. They also sell filters for the shower and bathtub, but unlike the carbon block or reverse osmosis filters, these filters only remove chlorine from the water.

Some people prefer to consume distilled water, but controversy exists over whether distilled water causes mineral deficiencies in the body. It may also be more expensive over the long run than purchasing a carbon block or reverse osmosis filter for the tap.

One disadvantage of carbon block filters is that they remove increasingly fewer contaminants over time, as the carbon gets used up. Some also remove a wider variety of pollutants than others. It pays to shop around to find a good one. One brand that I have used for years and which I highly recommend is Multipure, which removes many types of organic and inorganic pollutants. (The complete list of contaminants that these filters remove can be found at: www.multipure.com/mpscience).

In Summary

Nutrient deficiencies and toxic food are a primary cause of, or major contributing factor to, chronic illness experienced by people with tick-borne infections. Many studies have linked GMOs, pesticides, herbicides, heavy metals, preservatives and other toxic and artificial ingredients found in conventionally processed food to allergies, gastrointestinal dysfunction, autoimmune disease, cancer and other health problems. Conventionally processed food, in addition to containing many toxins, also has fewer nutrients than organic food, which makes it difficult for people with chronic illness who consume such food to obtain the nutrients that they need for recovery. This contributes to nutrient deficiencies in the chronically ill which exacerbates illness and makes recovery difficult. It is important to eat uncontaminated, fresh, natural and organic foods, and to take supplemental nutrients to make up for deficiencies in the body.

Chapter Three

Electromagnetic Radiation/Pollution

Electromagnetic radiation (EMR), emitted from sources ranging from Wi-Fi and cell phones to appliances, telecommunications towers, and power lines, is an underappreciated source of pollution in our environment. It is also a primary cause of, or contributing factor to, chronic illness involving tick-borne infections. Too much EMR exposure can block recovery from Lyme disease, as well as illness caused by mold and *Candida* infections, and other conditions of chronic illness. It may even be a primary cause of illness in some people, as I will demonstrate later in this chapter.

Electromagnetic radiation/pollution is invisible, and is usually not felt at the time of exposure. Many people thus mistakenly assume that it isn't a major factor in the development or furtherance of illness. Unfortunately, evidence about its damaging effects upon DNA, the immune system, and other parts of the body hasn't been widely published in the mainstream media (it can instead be found on sites such as www.bioinitiative.org). The U.S. government has also set extremely high limits for EMR exposure which far exceed what scientists who don't profit from EMR industries deem to be safe. For all of these reasons, people are falsely led to believe that this type of pollution isn't a big deal.

The telecommunications industry has also convinced people, through its advertising, that owning smartphones, cordless phones and Wi-Fi-enabled devices are a necessary and normal part of life. Exponential advances in the development of ever-more-attractive technological products make it difficult for people to turn away from these products, because they make their work and personal lives more productive, efficient, and financially profitable. The benefits of technology make it incredibly difficult for people to say "No" to their dangers.

This is true despite the fact that numerous studies indicate that the current levels of EMR to which most of us are exposed daily can damage the body, and even cause fatal illnesses such as cancer. These reports have been published in the scientific- and medical community-supported BioInitiative Report (www.bioinitiative.org); reputable journals such as the *American Journal of Industrial Medicine*; institutions such as the UCLA School of Public Health (www.ph.ucla.edu/pr/newsitem052108.html); and the World Health Organization (www.notowersnearschools.com/docs/20100520_flyer.pdf), to name just a few. The BioInitiative Report, which is compiled by an international working group of scientists, researchers, and public health policy professionals, has conducted over 2,000 studies on the damaging effects of EMR and is a valuable source of information for anyone concerned about its dangers.

Interestingly, whenever I talk to health-conscious people about the importance of eating organic food, avoiding chemical contaminants, and drinking clean water, they will agree with me. Yet when I talk to these same people about the importance of avoiding excessive electromagnetic radiation as part of maintaining wellness, they will look at me sideways or debate about how we need Wi-Fi and smartphones to survive in today's world. But EMR has been linked to cancer, autoimmune and other diseases. It can be just as dangerous as contaminated water, GMO food, or even infections.

In a May 2000 interview, the late orthopedic surgeon and Nobel Prize nominee Robert Becker, MD, who is also widely known as "the father of electromedicine" and author of *The Body Electric* and *Cross Currents*, stated, "I have no doubt in my mind that, at the present time, the greatest polluting element in the earth's environment is the proliferation of electromagnetic fields."

A few studies on the effects of EMR, especially from cell phones, have been published in the mainstream media. Unfortunately, most of these studies are sponsored by the telecommunications industry and are thus designed to result in outcomes that would favor the industry. George Carlo, PhD, JD, a medical scientist and epidemiologist who initiated the first telecommunications industry-backed studies on the dangers of cell phone use, stated in a 2007 *Life Extension* magazine article, "The Hidden Dangers of Cell Phone Radiation": "It's possible to design studies with pre-determined outcomes that still fall within the range of acceptable science. Thus, even highly flawed epidemiological studies can be published in peer-reviewed journals because they're judged against a pragmatic set of standards that assume the highest integrity among the investigators." The results of a study on cell phone dangers, which were published in the December 2006 edition of the *Journal of the National Cancer Institute*, concluded that cell phone use is safe. According to George Carlo, however, the results of this study were flawed, because the study was funded by the cell phone industry and designed to bring about a positive result.

It is difficult to participate in society without a cell phone, computer, Wi-Fi, and all the latest gadgets that make doing life and business easier. But it is also true that by exposing ourselves to excessive levels of EMR, we are conducting one of the greatest human experiments upon our health since the industrial revolution. While studies are already proving that EMR damages cells, causes cancer, and plays a role in other diseases such as Lyme and mold illness, we really have no idea about the full impact of its effects upon the body.

As a society, we haven't been exposed to high levels of EMR for a long enough period of time to determine just how severe the long-term effects will be. Also, disease can take years to develop following prolonged EMR exposure, which means that the full ramifications of current levels of EMR have yet to manifest in our bodies. For instance, the late Neil Cherry, PhD, former associate professor of Environmental Health at Lincoln University, wrote in his 2002 report "Epidemiological studies of enhanced Brain/CNS Cancer incidence and mortality from EMR and EMF exposures" that ". . . latency between beginning magnetic field exposures and diagnosis of adult cancer typically fell into the range [of] 4 to 9 years, peaking at 7 years to develop following EMR exposure." Thus, current cases of cancer that have been attributed to EMR may reflect exposure from several or more years ago, when EMR levels were much lower than they are now.

Today, one in two people is developing cancer. According to studies, some of these cancers have been linked largely, or in part, to EMR exposure. This means that as EMR levels continue to increase, the incidence of cancer and other diseases caused by EMR are likely to increase, as well. The amount of EMR in the environment is increasing significantly every year, as new telecom towers are constructed, Wi-Fi replaces hard-wired Internet connections, fluorescent lightbulbs replace incandescent lightbulbs, and so on. We are constructing for ourselves an incredibly dangerous environment in which to live.

Because people don't get sick from EMR right away (although some sensitive people can feel its effects immediately), and studies about its dangers have been ignored, downplayed, and denied in the media, most of society is walking around in a cloud of oblivion about its perilous effects upon the body. It's nice to save an hour during the day by talking on a cell or cordless phone while driving home from work, and our jobs may require us to utilize Wi-Fi technology in the office, but the cost of our more efficient lives may carry a tremendous price tag: the loss of our health.

In some Western European countries such as Switzerland, Austria, Germany, and Denmark, electromagnetic pollution is more widely recognized and accepted as a health hazard. According to information taken from a chart in the award-winning book, *Wireless Radiation Rescue,* by Kerry Crofton, PhD, safety standards for EMR exposure are much stricter in these countries. According to Dr. Crofton's research, even Russia and China have stricter standards for EMR exposure than the United States does!

Unfortunately, in the United States, safety standards are based on studies that have been conducted by scientists who have financial ties to the telecommunications industry. As previously noted, results from such studies are biased. Even when unbiased studies have been conducted, the results have been ignored by the government, perhaps because it receives so much of its tax revenue from the telecom industry. If the government were to actually acknowledge the dangers of EMR and set revised safety standards for EMR exposure, it would incur the loss of millions of dollars in revenue from the telecom industry. The dangers of EMR are mostly ignored by the powers that be.

Dr. Crofton's book also contains a chart of indoor EMR safety guidelines for the sleeping area, which are based on recommendations from the German Institut für Baubiologie und Ökologie Neubeuern (IBN), a group of building biology professionals who are dedicated to the development of safe standards of exposure to indoor environmental contaminants. Their recommendations are based on the results of studies that were conducted by unbiased scientists on the effects of indoor EMR exposure. According to the building biology scientists and Dr. Crofton's book, adverse affects to cells begin to occur when continual exposure to indoor magnetic fields exceeds 0.2 mG (milligauss). (Note: magnetic fields are measured in milligauss, while electric fields are often measured in V/m or µW/m2 [microwatts per square meter].)

When magnetic fields exceed 5 mG, severe effects to the body can occur. Yet, in North America, safety guidelines allow for the general public to be exposed to 833 mG on a continual basis, and for people who work in the telecom or related industries, to be exposed to 4,166 mG. And these are just the standards for magnetic fields. For radio frequency (RF) radiation exposure, the U.S. government has set the maximum allowed level at 2–10 million µW/m2. Yet safe limits of exposure are estimated by scientists to be around 0.1 microwatts per square meter. When continual exposure exceeds 1,000 microwatts, according to the building biologists, extremely damaging effects to cells can occur over time. Thus, the amount of radiation that we are exposed to is literally *millions* of times higher than what scientists who have studied the effects of EMR upon the body consider to be safe.

In addition, Dr. Crofton's book contains a chart that outlines different countries' limits and standards for radio frequency (RF) exposure from cell towers. For example, according to the chart, the Health Department in Salzburg, Austria, has set levels of safe RF exposure for the public at 1 µW/m2. Many other European countries, such as Belgium, France, and Germany, have set maximum exposure levels at anywhere from 1,000–2,500,000 µW/m2, depending upon the country and situation. Yet according to Dr. Crofton, the BioInitiative Working Group recommends that continual indoor exposure to RFs be no higher than 100 µW/m2. The U.S. government, meanwhile, allows a staggering 100,000,000 µW/

m2 of RF in the environment on a continual basis. Thus, the gap between what most unbiased scientists consider to be safe levels of EMR exposure and what the government allows is astronomical.

How Electromagnetic Radiation Damages the Body, and Why It May Be a Primary Cause of Illness in People with Chronic Lyme Disease

Electromagnetic radiation (EMR), by itself, can cause disease to the body, regardless of the other environmental pollutants that may also be affecting it. EMR can trigger symptoms in people who harbor tick-borne infections by weakening their immune function, but can also exacerbate infectious activity. Pathogenic growth is encouraged by constant levels of damaging high-frequency electromagnetic pollution. It also slows down the body's production of healthy bacteria, which defend against pathogens.

Thomas M. Rau, MD, of the renowned Swiss Paracelsus Clinic, stated in an interview that was transcribed online at www.emrstop.org, "We have more organisms than cells in our bodies. Cultures of normal human endogenous bacterial cultures grow much less when exposed to EMR. They grow less when they are around a mobile phone, a tower, or cordless phone." He then said, "Growing less good bacteria in your body means you will have an overgrowth of bad bacteria that can result in things like Lyme disease. Especially from the east coast of the USA, we have many patients with Lyme. Antibiotics only make it worse."

In his interview, Dr. Rau seems to imply that Lyme disease symptoms can result from EMR exposure, since EMR affects the body's ability to produce disease-fighting bacteria that would otherwise eliminate Lyme organisms or keep them in check. Perhaps EMR sensitivity isn't just a side effect of chronic illness or Lyme disease, but instead sets the stage for people to become ill from tick-borne organisms and other factors. If this is true, then EMR has profound implications for those with Lyme disease, because it means that people with Lyme don't suffer from symptoms just because they have Lyme. They suffer from Lyme because EMR weakens the immune system and causes infections to gain a foothold and flourish in the body. EMR may be, therefore, a primary or contributing factor to disease for some people, especially since ample evidence proves that EMR, by itself, is a powerful cell-altering and immune-altering toxin that causes disease, regardless of whether tick-borne infections are also present in the body.

According to the website, www.emrstop.org, 3,000 of the 10,000 patients that the Paracelsus Clinic sees annually suffer from symptoms of electromagnetic hypersensitivity. That is nearly one-third of its chronically ill! If one-third of the patients who attend a world-renowned clinic have symptoms of EMR sensitivity, imagine how many more will be impacted in the years to come, as EMR exposure increases.

Environmental EMR doesn't just encourage the growth of tick-borne infections. As I will discuss in Chapter Four, Mold and Mycotoxins, mold multiplies and produces more toxins in the presence of harmful EMR, and increases symptoms in people with mold toxicity. It is therefore more difficult for people with mold toxicity to recover in the presence of EMR. It is important not only for people with tick-borne infections, but also for those with mold, to reduce their exposure to EMR, if they are to fully recover.

Encouraging pathogenic growth isn't the only way in which EMR affects the body. Scientific studies have proven that even low levels of EMR (much less than what most of us are exposed to daily) damage DNA by generating free radicals and creating cell mutations that lead to cancer. Such studies can be found on EMR activist Camilla Rees' website, (www.electromagneti-chealth.org), in the BioInitiative Report mentioned earlier in this chapter, and within Dr. Cherry's reports: "Evidence that EMF/EMR causes Leukaemia/Lymphoma in Adults and Children" and "Epidemiological studies of enhanced Brain/CNS Cancer incidence and mortality from EMR and EMF exposures."

In addition to creating cell mutations and damaging DNA, electromagnetic pollution alters the body's ability to manufacture stress proteins, which play an integral role in immune function. It also disrupts the normal functioning of the neurological, cardiovascular, and endocrine systems, by altering intercellular and intracellular communication. As if that weren't enough, it disrupts the proper functioning of the blood-brain barrier, which separates the blood from the brain's extracellular fluid in the central nervous system. This barrier helps to keep toxins out of the brain, and nutrients in. Such disruption allows damaging toxins to enter the brain.

Many scientists and researchers have established and confirmed these findings. For instance, Dr. Crofton, in her book, *Wireless Radiation Rescue,* notes that Professor Cherry discovered that EMR confuses and damages the cells' signaling system, and in some cases, as with cell phone use, nearly drowns out the signals. Disruptions in cell signaling, Cherry learned, produces symptoms such as headaches, concentration difficulties, memory loss, dizziness, and nausea, and long-term diseases such as Alzheimer's, brain tumors, and depression. Other scientists and researchers, including those who have contributed to the BioInitiative Report, have confirmed the above-mentioned effects of EMR.

Dr. Becker's studies on EMR have been particularly significant. He was among the first researchers to discover that exposure to abnormal electromagnetic fields (from computers, power lines, satellites, microwaves, and so forth) creates a stress response in the body. He found that if this exposure was prolonged, an individual's immune function would decline to below normal levels and leave the person susceptible to infectious disease and cancer. All physiological reactions in the body occur first on an energetic level, then on a biochemical level. Whatever affects the body's energy consequently impacts its biochemistry. Therefore, if energetic communications are disrupted, then biochemical processes will also become dysfunctional. Because EMR affects the energy of the entire body, a wide variety of problems and symptoms can result from exposure to this invisible toxin. For instance, in addition to the aforementioned, EMR can cause all of the following symptoms and conditions:

- Fatigue
- Cognitive problems
- Digestive disorders
- Pain
- Trouble breathing
- Insomnia
- Muscle/joint pain

- Dehydration
- Anxiety, depression
- Muscle weakness
- Altered sugar metabolism
- Tremors
- Numbness
- Ringing in the ears
- Skin rashes
- High or low blood pressure
- Altered heart rate
- Diseases of the brain and nervous system, including ADD (attention deficit disorder), ADHD (attention deficit hyperactivity disorder), MS (multiple sclerosis), ALS (amyotrophic lateral sclerosis), and Parkinson's.

Ironically, all of the above conditions are also symptoms of Lyme disease. Is it possible that some people with Lyme disease are really suffering from symptoms of EMR? Could it be that EMR is a primary trigger for Lyme disease symptoms and/or chronic illness, or what keeps some people from attaining a full recovery from tick-borne infections? Based on the evidence, I believe so.

Finally, the effects of EMR are greatly exacerbated by the amount of heavy metals in the body. Heavy metals attract and act as antennas for EMR. This includes metal from dental amalgams and implants, but also heavy metals that accumulate in the tissues and organs from the environment. According to George Carlo, PhD, JD, in the November 2007 edition of the *Australasian Journal of Clinical Environmental Medicine*, heavy metals in the brain act as antenna receptors in an EMR environment, and EMR exacerbates the toxic effects of heavy metals by closing down cell membranes and trapping metals within cells.

Dominique Belpomme, an oncology professor at Paris-Descartes University and president of the French Association for Research in Therapeutics Against Cancer (www.artac.info), sees many patients who have "Electromagnetic Intolerance Syndrome." He contends that certain factors cause people to be more susceptible to this syndrome, among these, " . . .

dental amalgam(s) that behave like antennas capturing airwaves." People with dental amalgams and who have high levels of heavy metal toxicity and are exposed to excessive levels of EMR may be more susceptible to sickness and an exacerbation of symptoms from heavy metal toxicity, as well as from the EMR itself."

Sadly, many people (if not most) with Lyme disease don't just suffer from the effects of tick-borne infections. Their immune systems are battling a fierce cocktail of contaminants, the most insidious of which include EMR, mold, and heavy metals. Focusing excessively upon treating the tick-borne infections and ignoring these other major causative factors of disease may produce for some people only minor to moderate improvements in recovery.

It is possible to mitigate the impact of EMR upon the body, by avoiding and removing sources of EMR in the home and workplace, and by using protective shielding devices. Following are suggestions for reducing EMR in the home. For some people, implementing some or all of these measures will be important for attaining a full recovery. The relevance and role of EMR in illness, like all toxins, however, is different for every person.

Finally, it's important to note that not all EMR is harmful. Electromagnetic devices, such as Rife and biophoton machines, which are used to treat Lyme disease and other infections, kill harmful microorganisms. But the frequencies used to eliminate the pathogens involved in Lyme disease are different from those that encourage pathogenic growth and which harm the body. Also, the energy of electromagnetic devices is applied judiciously and for limited periods of time, while environmental EMR is constant.

Essential Strategies for Reducing Electromagnetic Pollution in the Home

1. Remove or reduce exposure to Wi-Fi Internet in the home and replace it with a hard-wired broadband connection instead. Having a wireless Wi-Fi router is like having a mini-antenna inside the home. According to Stan Hartman, Environmental Consultant for RadSafe in Boulder, Colorado, when people have Wi-Fi antennas inside a router on their desks, they are getting about the same amount of radiation as they would if they were 30 meters (90 feet)

or less away from the large outdoor antennas of a typical cell phone base station (though the Wi-Fi signal typically isn't as constant as a cell phone signal). Also, with Wi-Fi and cordless phones, the body is exposed to a continuous signal without reprieve.

2. Eliminate cordless phones, especially DECT (Digitally Enhanced Communications Technology) phones, which emit as much EMR as cell phones. They can also be more dangerous than cell phones because they emit radio frequencies throughout the day and night. Like Wi-Fi, having a DECT phone is like having a cell phone antenna in the home. It isn't convenient for most people in our busy society to use a corded phone all of the time, but getting a long cord to walk around the house with, so that you can talk while doing other activities, may make the option more attractive. Corded phones are becoming increasingly difficult to find in stores, so I recommend checking online sites such as eBay for a wider variety of phone options.

3. Use a cell phone infrequently. If it's impossible for you to do this, because you need a cell phone for work, for example, use the speaker phone option on the phone whenever you talk. Keep the cell phone away from your body (e.g., leave it on the passenger seat when driving, and leave it inside the car at your place of destination). Turn it off if you plan to carry it with you. Most people carry cell phones inside their pockets or near their bodies in a purse, which is extremely dangerous. A lot of radiation exposure can be avoided by turning the phone off while carrying it around. Using a cell phone in a car is especially dangerous, since the metal in the car amplifies the effects of the radiation, and stronger signals are required to maintain a constant connection in a moving vehicle. Not to mention the fact that more car accidents occur as a result of cell phone use!

Also, avoid using Bluetooth or wired headsets, both of which directly deliver radio frequencies to the head. Studies have revealed Bluetooth wireless headsets to be more dangerous than other types of headsets. Joseph Mercola, DO, author of the world's most visited natural health site, www.mercola.com, writes in an online article,

"Does Your Cell Phone Fall at the Bottom of the Heap for Safety?": "Bluetooth wireless headsets are even worse than regular ones. Why? Because the wire is replaced with a transmitter and receiver, operating with low power at frequency levels between 900 MHz to 2.4 GHz. The maximum frequencies for wireless products compliant with Bluetooth specifications are 2.497 GHz. The frequency power of wireless headsets rivals that of microwave ovens, which also operate at 2.4 GHz."

Whenever cell phones are used, and regardless of how they are used—on speaker phone, with a headset, or with a Bluetooth device—the body is exposed to radiation, if not to the head then to whatever parts of the body the phone is closest to. Therefore, cell phones shouldn't be used for prolonged conversations, and ideally, not at all. It's also a good idea to keep the phone turned off when at home, since it constantly emits signals, even in standby mode.

The results of a recent study published on Camilla Rees' website, www.electromagnetichealth.org, revealed that just two and a half hours of monthly cell phone use dramatically increases the risk of developing gliomas, a type of brain cancer. Another study, published in Dr. Crofton's book, revealed that just a half hour of daily cell phone use over a period of ten years increases the risk of brain cancer by 140 percent. Excessive cell phone use has been linked, time and again, to brain cancer.

4. Choose a landline over Skype or other communications that involve attaching a headset to your computer. Computers emit very high levels of EMR, which are transferred through the headsets that plug into them. Whenever I use a headset with Skype, I become tired and mentally slow, after just a thirty-minute conversation. I have also found the radiation levels from using a headset with Skype to rival that of cordless and cell phones. Talking directly into the computer (if you have a newer computer) for Skype phone calls is a better idea. Using a landline is, of course, the best option.

5. Purchase a Faraday cage, a metallic-lined mesh net that drapes over the bed and which shields out 99 percent of all high-frequency EMR from the bed during sleep. (Note: high-frequency EMR is

that which comes from Wi-Fi, cell phone, and other sources of microwave and radio frequency radiation). Owning a Faraday cage is especially important if you live in an apartment, condominium, or townhome, and have neighbors above, beneath, and directly adjacent to you, each with his/her own Wi-Fi and cell phone network. Additionally, it's important that the bed be completely enclosed in metallic-lined material. Fabric that can be spread across the underside of the bed can be purchased separately from the Faraday cage. Some companies that sell these cages may provide the option of purchasing metallic fabric to line the underside of the bed, as well.

Whether or not you live in an apartment or townhome, however, most cities and towns nowadays, regardless of size, are blanketed in EMR, especially from Wi-Fi and cell phone towers, and everyone is exposed to it. People living in apartment-like situations may be exposed to higher levels because they have more neighbors with Wi-Fi in their immediate vicinity. Unfortunately, not everyone can afford to live in a house, or away from crowded cities (where most jobs are), so using a Faraday cage at night can compensate for some of the exposure to high-frequency EMR. Protecting the body from EMR at night is especially important because the body repairs and regenerates itself during sleep. EMR interferes with this process. That said, a Faraday cage won't protect the body from low-frequency sources of EMR, such as electrical appliances and wiring. It's also a good idea to turn off the circuit breakers in the house at night and unplug all electronics in the bedroom.

Environmental consultant Stan Hartman of RadSafe provided the following information about Faraday cages in an email to me:

"A Faraday cage (a grounded metallic cage or curtain) will be effective for keeping out electric fields and radio frequencies (including microwave radiation from cell phones, Wi-Fi, radio/TV broadcasts, radar, etc.), but it won't keep out low-frequency alternating magnetic fields, such as from power lines, bad wiring, etc. If you get two meters (a Gauss and 3-axis RF Field Strength meter), you can easily check to see how well the cage shields you. If it completely encloses the bed (including underneath) it should shield you from electric fields and RF, but not magnetic fields. If it doesn't completely enclose the bed, though, any metal within the cage—especially long, straight metal—can pick up RF & microwave radiation and re-radiate it. That's the problem with shielding—it can either work well or possibly make things worse—which is why it's good to have a meter to check with."

To avoid attracting electromagnetic energy into the Faraday cage, it's also important to avoid metal bed frames and to sleep on a futon, air, wool or other non-metal-containing mattress.

(More on EMR meters will be described in the following pages).

6. Sleep on Earthing sheets (www.earthinginstitute.net), and place an Earthing mat under your feet while you work at the computer. Earthing involves connecting the body to the earth through various grounding techniques. It is one way to normalize the body's energy. Earthing provides electrons to the body (in the same way that antioxidant nutrients provide electrons to the body, and quench free radicals). A metallic-lined sheet (usually carbon or silver-lined) is connected to a grounding cord, which is then plugged into the round opening below the two vertical prongs on an electrical outlet or connected directly into the ground via a grounding rod. Electrons from the earth then get transferred to the sheet, and subsequently, to whatever is in contact with that sheet. Lying on an Earthing sheet therefore causes these electrons to get transferred to the body, where they balance its electrical system. As a result, the body becomes less impacted by harmful EMR.

Some people believe that Earthing completely blocks the harmful effects of EMR, but I don't know whether I agree, since I still suffer from symptoms of electromagnetic pollution whenever I spend extended periods of time at my computer, even when I place my barefoot feet on an Earthing mat. If you sleep on Earthing sheets, be aware that aligning the body's energy can provoke a detoxification reaction at first, which can last several weeks. I experienced this when I first began sleeping on my Earthing sheets, but I also began to sleep more deeply as a result of the sheets. It is possible to minimize the undesirable symptoms of spontaneous detoxification that can occur with Earthing by Earthing for only short periods of time at first; say, for 15 minutes or an hour at a time.

Standing or sitting barefoot on the ground outside also normalizes the body's energy field. It can be healing to spend several hours outdoors with your feet on the earth. For more information on Earthing products, visit: www.earthinginstitute.net.

7. Do a search on www.antennasearch.com to discover how many microwave towers and antennas are within a four-mile radius of where you live. This can give you an idea of how much "outside" EMR you are exposed to. It's not uncommon for high-density urban areas to have 50 or more towers, and over 150 antennas within a four-mile radius. Through my searches on www.antennasearch.com, I have discovered that most suburbs in the Denver area, where I used to live, have approximately 25-35 towers, but some areas have 50 or more. In the small town where I now live, there are only four towers within a four-mile radius of my condominium.

While it's a good idea to know how many towers are near your home, it's also important to bear in mind that not all EMR towers and antennas are created equal. Some emit stronger fields than others, or emit radiation more consistently than others. It can be difficult to generalize about safe distances; many variables factor into the amount of EMR that towers produce. Towers also have different numbers of antennas, which all have a different geometry, angle, and amount of "traffic" that they are servicing.

The best way to determine outdoor EMR levels, in addition to doing a tower and antenna search, is by purchasing an EMR meter that measures electrical and/or magnetic fields. Stan Hartman recommends a gaussmeter for detecting the low-frequency magnetic fields that come from power lines, household appliances, and bad wiring in the home. One decent product is the ElectroSensor, which can be found at www.lessemf.com/gauss.html; however, this meter is probably better for people who aren't extremely electrosensitive. As Stan Hartman points out, the readings on cheaper gaussmeters aren't always completely accurate. If a gaussmeter is off in its reading by even half a milligauss, that could matter to an extremely electrosensitive person. According to Hartman, some electrosensitive people can tolerate exposure to 1.5 mG, but not to 2 mG. He contends that the least expensive, yet accurate gaussmeter is the Single Axis Digital AC Gaussmeter/Teslameter, which costs approximately $80.00. It's important to know how to use this type of meter. It can give misleadingly low readings if improperly used. For more information about how to use this meter, see Stan Hartman's instructions at: http://emfsafetystore.com/#meters.

When I asked Stan which meter he recommends for measuring radio/microwave radiation, he responded, "It's a bit more complicated for (measuring) radio frequencies—there really aren't any inexpensive meters that are accurate. The least expensive one I can recommend, considering its features and usefulness, is the first one listed on [the website] www.lessemf.com/rf.html, called the '3-Axis RF Meter.' It will give you a good idea of exposure levels to higher-frequency radiation—cell phones, cordless phones, Wi-Fi, etc." He went on to say, however, that, "This meter won't detect lower-frequency radiation from sources such as AM broadcasts and ham radio, and other things in the kilohertz range. It also won't detect extremely high-frequency sources like radar and some cordless phones [the ones labeled 5.8 GHz]. Accurate meters that cover a broad range like that cost thousands of dollars."

I purchased both a 3-axis RF Field Strength Meter and gaussmeter based on Stan's recommendations, and used both to help me find an area of suitable, low-EMR housing when I moved in 2011. These two tools, when used together, can provide a pretty good reading on the levels of low-frequency and high-frequency radiation in the environment, although the measurements that they provide are not exact. Extremely electrosensitive people may want to invest in more expensive meters or find an environmental consultant to help them determine the EMR levels in their home and workplace.

8. If you live close to major power lines, move. According to a study that was published in the June 2005 edition of the *British Medical Journal*, researchers found that children who lived within

650 feet of a power line had a 70 percent greater risk for leukemia than children who lived 2,000 feet away or more.

Scientists who study the effects of EMR upon the body believe that high-voltage power lines should not be constructed anywhere near to where people work or live. Use a gaussmeter to estimate how much radiation you are exposed to from these lines. If you discover that your home is within range of dangerous EMR fields, and you aren't able to move, consider painting all of your walls and doors with EMR shielding paint, and covering the windows with metal screening or shielding fabric. More information about these shielding products and how to use them can be found at The EMF Safety SuperStore: http://www.lessemf.com/paint.html.

9. Get rid of your microwave. Besides emitting dangerous high-fre-quency EMR, microwaves alter the molecular configuration of food, rendering it carcinogenic.

10. According to Dr. Croften, baby monitors emit high levels of wireless and digital microwave radiation that can affect a baby's development. If you have a baby, don't use one of the newer baby monitors on the market. Crofton recommends using an older type of monitor, which doesn't rely on digital or wireless technology, and placing it at least six feet away from the baby.

11. Use only LED or incandescent light bulbs in your home, instead of the newer energy-saving fluorescent light bulbs. The new bulbs emit extremely high levels of electromagnetic radiation. (I'm afraid, though, that by the time this book is published, incandescent bulbs may no longer be available at retail stores. Hopefully you can still find them secondhand on eBay or through other online stores). LED bulbs are also safe to use, and are more efficient than incan-descent light bulbs. They are more readily available, but they are also more expensive.

12. Minimize the amount of metal furniture in your home and workplace. Metal acts as an antenna for EMR. If you use a Faraday cage to filter out EMR from your sleeping environment, it's especially important to make sure that the cage isn't draped over a bed that has metal

springs, a metal frame, or even metal coils. These can attract EMR and trap it inside the cage, thereby potentially increasing, rather than decreasing, the amount of radiation within! Radio frequencies are attracted to metal and travel along it.

13. Remove all dental amalgams and metal sources from your body, including heavy metal toxins that may have accumulated there from environmental sources. (More information on heavy metal chelation can be found in Chapter Five). Heavy metals attract radiation to the body and act as transmitters for EMR, thus exacerbating symptoms of both heavy metal and EMR toxicity.

14. If you work at a computer during the day, or your occupation involves excessive exposure to EMR (which is the case for most of us), consider purchasing EMR-protective clothing. The EMF Safety SuperStore, www.lessemf.com, has a few good products, including an EMR apron that can be easily taken on and off every day. Other shielding fabrics and products can be found at: www.emfsafetystore.com.

15. Consider purchasing EMR-shielding material for your computer screen to protect your eyes from the effects of EMR and UV radiation. Other types of shielding material exist for computers; I personally have not found any that fully protect the body from the effects of the powerful EMR that they emit. Some products may be helpful for reducing exposure, although extensive studies haven't been done on most of them. Their benefits are uncertain.

16. Consider "destructive interference." Recently, I have been made aware of a new type of technology that may completely protect the body from the damaging effects of radiation from computers, as well as all other devices and sources of both low- and high-frequency radiation. This technology, invented by the German engineer Winfried M. Dochow and upon which the German company Memon was founded, is based upon a principle called "destructive interference." This technique is described on the Memon website (www.memonyourharmony.com):

"In nature too, there are not only positive vibrations, but also ones whose information quality can have a damaging effect in the long term. These include vibrations from underground water veins and rock faults. The memon® transformers can completely delete the damaging information waves from all vibration fields (static, electromagnetic, electric or pulsed) using the process of destructive interference. This means that two waves of the same wavelength, frequency, speed, phase and amplitude meet one another. If these waves are also 180° out from one another in terms of phase (the trough of one wave meets the crest of another and vice versa), then the two waves cancel each other out. This phenomenon is known as destructive interference."

Memon's transformer products, when placed on an appliance or device such as a cell phone or power strip, cancel out the deleterious effects of the radiation emitted from these devices. Unlike other types of EMR technology, which block or shield the body from radiation, memon technology transforms and harmonizes the behavior of the radiation so that it ceases to be harmful to the body.

According to Ferry Hirschmann's book, *The Memon Revolution*, Dochow tested this technology on thousands of people before creating Memon. Testimonials and the results of studies proving its benefits can be found on the Memon website. This technology has been available in Germany since at least 2001. It has just recently begun to be promoted in the United States. Memon makes transformer products for the car, cell phone, computer (and other devices) as well as a memonizerCOMBI, which protects the entire house from both high-frequency and low-frequency radiation. For more information on Memon and its transformer products, visit: www.memonyourharmony.com.

17. Limit the use of appliances, whenever possible. Portable fans and air conditioners, if they are run continuously, can be particularly harmful sources of low-frequency EMR.

18. Purchase Graham-Stetzer filters, which remove or reduce the effects of electricity and electrical wiring in the walls of your home or office. Most of this type of radiation falls within the radio frequency (RF) range and radiates dangerous EMR several feet into the room,

even when all electricity and electrical devices are turned off. For more information on these filters, visit: www.stetzerelectric.com. Several studies have proven these filters to improve symptoms of disease in some people.

Finally, it's important to note that not all EMR products are reputable or helpful, and some may counteract the effects of others. It's important to consult with an EMR expert before employing multiple strategies to reduce EMR in the home. Some EMR products negatively impact the body's energetic field, rather than protect it. I don't understand all of the reasons for this, but some EMR-protective devices, whether worn on the body or placed on an appliance or other source of EMR (such as a computer or cell phone), aren't always beneficial. Not many scientific studies have been conducted on these types of devices, so proof of their effectiveness is limited. For instance, some people have told me that they feel better when they wear pendants designed to block EMR, while others claim that they feel worse. Still others note only temporary benefits that seem to wear off over time. Personally, I have wasted hundreds of dollars on EMR products such as pendants and USB devices for my computer. They don't seem to have delivered what they promised. I felt no different as a result of using them, and instead remained sensitive to the EMR that they were supposed to protect me from. It can be difficult to determine whether protective devices are effective. Negative reactions to such devices may be caused by a detoxification process, which gets set in motion by the device, and occurs when the body's energy field becomes properly aligned. But negative reactions can also be due to the device negatively impacting the person's energy field, or simply failing to provide any protective benefit at all.

I don't endorse the use of any type of energy-protecting or blocking gadgets, appliances, or devices, other than those mentioned in this chapter. I don't believe that enough studies have been done on them to determine their effectiveness. In general, removing sources of EMR or avoiding exposure to EMR is a more reliable and effective strategy for protecting the body against harmful electromagnetic pollution than trying to combat it with protective devices.

(Note: I receive no financial or other compensation for mentioning any of the EMR-protective products in this chapter).

In Summary

Electromagnetic pollution may be a primary or perpetuating cause of symptoms in people with tick-borne infections and chronic illness. It is therefore crucial to reduce EMR exposure and protect the body, workplace, and home against its damaging effects. Reducing EMR exposure also enables the body to mount a more effective immune response against pathogens, by preserving healthy bacterial growth, inter- and intracellular communications, and other aspects of immune function. Reducing EMR can prevent tick-borne infections from causing symptoms, and may prevent recurrences of symptoms in those who have already been treated for infections.

Chapter Four

Mold and Mycotoxins

Increasingly, Lyme-literate healthcare practitioners are finding that mold and the toxins that they produce (called mycotoxins) are a major cause of symptoms in their patients with Lyme disease. Mold toxicity results when a genetically susceptible or immune-compromised person is exposed for a prolonged period of time to the interior of a water-damaged motor vehicle or building. The mold and mycotoxins that are found in such environments infect and cause illness in those who inhabit them.

According to biotoxin expert Ritchie Shoemaker, MD, approximately one-quarter of the population has a genetic inability to eliminate mold, mycotoxins, and other biotoxins from their bodies. In people with chronic illness, that percentage is probably much higher. The people who can't eliminate mold and mycotoxins aren't effectively making antibodies to mold, and the toxins they produce. Instead, their bodies allow the fungi and the associated toxins to remain in their tissues and organs, where they can wreak havoc for years, undetected by the immune system. If such people are continually exposed to mold, they will become more and more ill until they are able to do an aggressive mold detoxification protocol.

Mold toxicity isn't an incidental problem in people with Lyme disease. Sometimes, it is a primary cause of illness that may be even more salient in the overall symptom picture than tick-borne infections. While tick-borne infections create immune dysfunction that may make people susceptible to sickness from mold and the toxins they produce, mold and mycotoxins can also make people susceptible to symptoms from tick-borne infections.

Lisa Nagy, MD, a mold toxin survivor and Lyme-literate doctor, stated in an interview with me that environmental factors (such as food allergies, hormonal problems, toxicity from pesticides, etc.) are often what really cause or instigate symptoms in people with Lyme disease. She cites mold as being one of these factors, and contends that mold damages the immune system and renders people unable to effectively fight tick-borne infections. In people with both Lyme and mold toxicity, symptoms may not be caused primarily by Lyme, but rather by mold and other environmental factors. Dr. Nagy also contends that environmental illness predisposes people to symptoms from tick-borne infections. Most Lyme disease patients should also be assessed for mold and other environmental toxins. She believes that some Lyme-literate doctors get stuck in a false mentality that a single offending agent (tick-borne infections) is the main cause of disease in people with Lyme. She says that they must instead address all environmental causes of disease, including mold. Dr. Nagy notes that mold is so prevalent in our society that the Environmental Health Center of Dallas (www.ehcd.com) found that 60 percent of the environmentally ill people who came to its clinic had mold toxicity as a primary cause of their symptoms.

Symptoms of Mold Toxicity and How Mold Damages the Body

Mold and the toxins that they produce (mycotoxins) cause inflammation. They damage multiple organs and systems, as the body attacks its own tissues through an exaggerated and ongoing pro-inflammatory cytokine response. (Cytokines are substances secreted by the immune system that have an effect on the other cells in the body). Often, this cytokine response continues even after the offending toxins are removed from the body. When people are initially exposed to mold, they may experience any of the following mold allergy symptoms:

- Sneezing
- Skin redness, itchiness, and irritation
- Watery, itching eyes
- Headaches

People who are able to effectively detoxify mold and its mycotoxins will experience these symptoms for only as long as they are in a moldy environment. The other 25 percent will go on to develop more severe chronic symptoms, due to their bodies' inability to remove mold and mycotoxins. The longer a person is exposed to a moldy environment, the more severe the symptoms he or she will experience. Such symptoms include, but aren't limited to:

- Fatigue
- Weakness
- Confusion
- Numbness
- Tingling
- Tremors
- Increased urination
- Excessive thirst
- Mood swings
- Sweats (especially night sweats)
- Light sensitivity
- Shortness of breath
- Stiffness
- Memory problems
- Red eyes
- Aches and pains
- Cough, sinus problems
- Headaches
- Concentration problems
- Joint Pain
- Abdominal pain
- Muscle cramps

People with mold toxicity, like those with Lyme disease, can present with a wide variety of symptoms which overlap with those of tick-borne infections. For this reason, it can sometimes be difficult to ascertain whether symptoms are due primarily to Lyme disease or to mold toxins. Many people have both, and treating mold toxicity and the inflammatory responses that it causes shouldn't be an afterthought. Also, it can be just as difficult and challenging to eliminate mold and heal from the immune system damage that it causes as it can be to heal from tick-borne infections. Both tick-borne infections and mold must be treated. It isn't true that treating tick-borne infections will enable the body to get rid of mold and mold toxins on its own (unlike some opportunistic viruses). It may not be possible for the body to heal from tick-borne infections unless mold and mold toxins are also removed from the body and the corresponding inflammatory responses they cause are addressed.

Lab Tests That Detect Mold in the Body As Well As the Home

When diagnosing mold toxicity, healthcare practitioners should evaluate several factors, including their patients' symptoms and history of exposure to water-damaged buildings, along with a variety of lab test markers. Many people who are sick from mold and mycotoxins have negative lab test results. Lab tests don't exist for all the types of mold and mold toxins that are present in water-damaged buildings. So while tests for these toxins are useful, they have their limitations.

RealTime Laboratories may be one of the more effective labs for mycotoxin testing. RealTime tests for three categories (not types) of mold toxins: tricothecenes, ochratoxins, and aflatoxins. Following is a description of each type of toxin and its dangers, according to data from the RealTime website (www.realtimelab.com):

Tricothecenes are mycotoxins produced by fungi such as *Stachybotrys* and *Fusarium*. They have the ability to kill healthy cells and can be very dangerous. These toxins are found in mold-infested buildings. The buildings' occupants get sick from inhaling their spores.

Ochratoxins are mycotoxins produced by fungi such as *Aspergillus ochraceus* and *Penicillium verrucosum, which are found in contaminated food*. These types of toxins aren't known to spread through the air. Instead, they're ingested along with moldy food. These molds usually grow on improperly stored food and/or food that has been stored for too long. They are most often found in grain and pork products, but can also be found in coffee and on fruits.

Aflatoxins are mycotoxins produced by a wide variety of *Aspergillus* species. The most common aflatoxins are produced by *Aspergillus flavus* and *Aspergillus parasiticus*. They are very toxic and can cause cancer. High-level aflatoxin exposure also damages the liver and causes liver cirrhosis and liver failure.

RealTime Labs tests for the above-mentioned mycotoxins through antibody and DNA tests, using tissue, saliva, and urine samples. They can also test for mold in the work and home environment.

Another useful type of test for measuring mold levels in the home is the ERMI^{SM} DNA mold test. ERMI stands for Environmental Relative Moldiness Index, which measures the presence and concentrations of over 36 mold species in the home, based on a sample of dust. The ERMI test was developed by scientists at the Environmental Protection Agency. Free home-testing kits can be obtained at www.ermimoldtest.com.

Molds vary in the severity of their effects upon the body. Some mold toxins aren't toxic to humans, or are toxic at only very high levels. Thus, sending in a sample of dust from the home or workplace to a laboratory may help to determine whether a particular mold is causing symptoms of toxicity. Laboratory technicians can indicate which molds are toxic to the body and which aren't, if you ask them. Once mold exposure has been confirmed, a diagnosis of mold toxicity can be made by testing the body for mold and mycotoxins, evaluating a variety of inflammatory markers, and analyzing symptoms. Inflammatory markers that indicate the possible presence of mycotoxins and other biotoxins are described later in this chapter.

The Prevalence of Mold in the Home and Workplace

Some people don't give mold and mycotoxins more than a passing thought because they can't see or smell mold in their homes and therefore conclude that they don't have a mold problem. Yet mold cannot always be detected by a visual or odor inspection. Mold may be present even in the absence of musty smells, high levels of humidity, and water leaks. The best way to detect and determine whether mold is present in your environment is to send a dust sample to one of the aforementioned laboratories, and have a mold remediation expert inspect your home (if mold is suspected based on the lab test). It is likewise important to test cars and any other interior environment that you are exposed to on a regular basis.

Research suggests that mold is more prevalent in homes than most people realize. Richard Loyd, PhD, a nutritionist who helps many of the chronically ill to recover their health, writes in a mold article that he distributes to his clients: "Researchers at Harvard University studied 5000 homes and found that fully half of them had enough mold toxins in them to cause symptoms. The situation is similar in most parts of the country. Almost half of the people in the USA are living in homes that have enough mold toxins to make them sick to some degree."

In his "Mold Toxins Summary" article, found at: www.royalrife.com, Dr. Loyd writes that concrete that is in contact with dirt wicks moisture and is a continual source of water vapor. Any natural fibers such as wood or sheetrock paper that are exposed to this moisture will harbor mold spores. If your house is built on a concrete slab or has an attached garage or basement, it may have mold. Dr. Loyd contends that almost all cars are moldy, even new ones. This is because moisture from snow and rain often gets inside cars and creates a hospitable environment where mold can grow. For most people, having a bit of mold in the home isn't a problem. But for the 25 percent of the population whose bodies don't properly eliminate mold and its toxins (which is also many of the chronically ill), even the slightest exposure to mold may cause symptoms.

Mold Remediation for the Home

If you suspect that you have severe water damage to your home, it is a good idea to call a mold remediation expert to ascertain whether mold is present, and if so, have it removed. If the damage to your home has been severe, it may be necessary to move. According to Dr. Loyd, if your home or car doesn't smell musty or have extensive water damage, mold spores can sometimes be removed by diffusing essential oils throughout the home environment with a cold air diffuser. Diffusers use compressed air to disperse oil throughout the room in the form of a fine mist. Thieves

Essential Oil Blend (www.secretofthieves.com) is one product that is often used for this purpose. Dr. Loyd also makes an essential oil concoction for removing mold called Detox Oil, which he believes is even more effective than Thieves oil. It contains essential oils of cloves, lemon, cinnamon, eucalyptus, and rosemary, as well as bee propolis, and can be purchased at www.royalrife.com.

Diffusing or dispersing essential oils throughout every room in the home with a cold air diffuser for 24–72 hours kills mold spores. However, a few spores always remain after every "essential oil bath," according to Dr. Loyd. It is therefore necessary to diffuse the home on a monthly basis, for 24 hours per room, and to diffuse cars more frequently.

The only problem with using essential oils to remove mold is that when they kill mold, they may cause even more mycotoxins to be released into the environment. When mold dies, it releases toxins. Also, the essential oils can kill mold in the body and cause a Herxheimer (detoxification) reaction, as the molds release mycotoxins into the body. Thus, it may be feasible to diffuse your living environment with essential oils only if you can spend several days away from your home or the building that is being treated.

If you choose to use a cold-air diffuser to remove mold, it's important to know that not all cold-air diffusers work well for this purpose. Some require that water be added to them, and don't allow sufficient concentrations of oil to be distributed throughout the environment. Others are inefficient. One good brand of diffuser that I recommend is the Aroma-Pro Essential Air Diffuser, which can be purchased at www.DiffuserWorld.com.

Ozone generators also remove mold from the environment. Ozone may be a better choice than essential oils, as doctors such as Lee Cowden, MD, have found that people who use essential oils on a regular basis may eventually develop sensitivities or allergies to them. On the other hand, some authorities advise against using ozone air purifiers, as some studies have shown that they can harm the lungs and immune system. As with essential oils, ozone may be a more viable option if you can avoid being on-site during the mold cleanup period.

Besides these two do-it-yourself remedies, the only other way to remove mold from the environment—and probably the safest and most effective way to do it—is to call in a mold remediation expert. These experts can detect mold in places that the eye can't see, such as behind walls and beneath carpeting. Remediation experts remove materials that have been contaminated by mold, including wall material, insulation, flooring, carpet, and cabinetry. They also treat the contaminated area with mildicide and other mold-killing substances, and correct and remove the source of water damage. If the damage is extensive and severe, however, it may be necessary to vacate the mold-affected environment permanently.

When detoxifying the home or workplace of mold, it is also essential to get rid of all clothes, books, bedding, and furniture that smell musty, sweet, or pungent, or which are discolored. Strange smells and discoloration all indicate mold. Getting a high-efficiency particulate (HEPA) air filter for the bedroom and/or other rooms in the house to mop up airborne toxins is also a good idea, as is keeping all potentially moldy books and magazines out of the sleeping area. Austin Air and Nikken make high-quality air filters. Because mold flourishes in carpet, replacing the carpet with some type of hard-surface flooring may also be necessary. Ceramic tile is ideal.

My Personal Experience with Mold Toxicity

A sales clerk at an auto parts store once informed me that mold was the reason for the musty smell coming from my car's air conditioning system. When I cleaned out the air conditioner, the musty smell disappeared. But a car or building doesn't have to smell musty or have visible mold in order to be contaminated.

Until recently, I assumed that my condominium wasn't moldy, since it's fairly new, hasn't had any water leaks, and doesn't smell musty. Besides, I live in one of the driest states in the country—Colorado. And until recently, no doctor had ever told me that mold toxins were playing a role in my symptom picture. Yet testing on a ZYTO biocommunication machine, along with a saliva test, revealed that my body was harboring high amounts of mold toxins. I was surprised, but then recalled that in years past, I have lived in homes where water leaks were common. I also lived in Costa Rica for two years, where it rains nine months out of the year. In Costa Rica, it is nearly impossible to live in a home that doesn't have some mold. Because I never felt worse in these places, I assumed that mold wasn't a problem for me. I was wrong!

The moral of this story is that it's always best to test your home or work environment to determine whether mold is present. Don't rely upon a musty smell! It's also important to consider your lifelong history of exposure to water-damaged buildings when determining whether mold might be a factor in your symptom picture.

Mold Treatments for the Body

Healing from mold-induced illness involves not only removing mold and its mycotoxins from the body, and remediating water-damaged buildings, but also lowering the pro-inflammatory cytokine responses that mold and its toxins can cause. More information about restoring immune function and normalizing cytokine response is described at the end of this chapter.

When removing mold from the body, it's important to note that separate treatments are needed for mold and for their mycotoxins. Mold is a live organism (a fungi). It must be eliminated using antimicrobial remedies, and its toxins removed with powerful toxin binders. Banderol and Cumanda, products made by NutraMedix (www.nutramedix.com) are effective at killing fungi, as are olive leaf extract and many other herbs, including clove, cinnamon, peppermint, and rosemary. These are among some of the strongest antifungal remedies.

MMS, or Miracle Mineral Supplement, has also been proven in patient case studies to have powerful antifungal properties. When mixed with citric acid or lemon juice, it produces chlorine dioxide, which has antimicrobial effects. However, this product should be used with extreme caution, as some doctors whom I have interviewed have found it to have unacceptable side effects. It should only be used under the guidance of a healthcare practitioner who is thoroughly familiar with its properties and effects upon the body.

It's also important to bind and remove the toxins that mold produces. Not just any toxin binder will suffice for this purpose. One of the most powerful and effective toxin binders is the cholesterol-lowering drug, cholestyramine. Cholestyramine binds to bile in the gall bladder and prevents any fat-soluble toxins contained in the gall bladder from re-circulating throughout the body. Cholestyramine is a drug and can cause side effects, especially in those who already have low cholesterol levels. For some, a better toxin binder choice might be activated carbon, or CholestePure, a natural plant-sterol-based product. That said, studies have shown this substance to be somewhat less effective. Dr. Loyd recommends CholestePure to his clients. He has also found that ionic footbaths help his clients recover from mold toxicity. In his article "Mold and Lyme Toxins," he describes how to make an inexpensive ionic footbath at home. This article can be found at: www.royalrife.com/mold_toxins.pdf.

James Schaller, MD, a Lyme-literate doctor and author of many books on tick-borne infections and mold, cites on his website the results of a study in which the effectiveness of four different types of widely used mold toxin binders was compared: www.usmoldphysician.com/articles/comparing-moldtoxinbinders.html. Of the four types of toxin binders that were studied, cholestyramine was shown to have the greatest capacity to absorb a certain type of mold toxin in the body. It was quite effective, having an 85 percent rate of absorption. Activated carbon had the second-highest rate of mold toxin absorption, at 62 percent. Bentonite clay was found to be only minimally effective, having a maximum absorption rate of 12 percent. In spite of its potential side effects, cholestyramine appears to be one of the best mold toxin binders on the market. Again, for those concerned about side effects, activated carbon or CholestePure may be a good second choice.

Activated carbon binds pharmaceutical drugs, herbs and nutrients that are in the gut. For that reason, it's important to ingest this substance as far away as possible (during the course of a day) from all other nutritional supplements, herbs and other remedies.

Dietary Recommendations

Maintaining a proper diet is important for reducing the impact of mold upon the body. It is essential to avoid moldy foods and foods that encourage inflammation. These include starchy, sugary, high-carbohydrate foods (including grains), and high-glycemic fruits. Some nightshade vegetables, such as tomatoes, may encourage mold growth, as will cheese, vinegar and alcoholic beverages.

It's also important to avoid consuming improperly stored food. Some foods are quick to grow mold on them, with mold spores present before you can even see them. When in doubt, don't store cooked food for more than 24 hours after the day it is prepared. This includes meat and cooked grains. I was surprised when energetic testing once revealed that my brown rice had mold on it just two days after I had cooked it—even though no mold was visible on the rice, and it still tasted good.

Nuts tend to grow mold on them, as do cured and smoked meats. Soaking nuts in lemon juice or baking them in the oven may remove the spores. Peanuts and peanut butter should be avoided entirely, as they often harbor mold, even when stored in the refrigerator. Other nuts and nut butters should be stored in the refrigerator.

The Synergistic Effects of Mold, Heavy Metals, and Electromagnetic Radiation

One well-respected Lyme-literate doctor (whose name I must withhold for privacy purposes), has found that mold harbors toxic heavy metals, at the same time that it protects the body from their effects. When doing a mold and mold toxin removal protocol, it may also be a good idea to take some heavy metal binding agents. Heavy metals sometimes get released into the body when mold is killed off. If these metals are released too quickly, and no binders are available to carry them out of the body, they can get redistributed into the tissues and organs, where they can then cause further damage to the body.

I discovered this for myself, the hard way. Once I learned that my body harbored mold, I began to use Banderol to eliminate it. As a result, a massive flood of heavy metals was released from the mold into my bloodstream. Since heavy metals act as conductors, or antennas, for electromagnetic fields (EMFs), I concurrently became extremely sensitive to EMFs. I began to experience weakness in my right arm and leg, and feelings of anxiety, which were exacerbated every time I used my cell phone or sat in front of my computer. Since then, eliminating the metals has been a difficult task and I have had to limit my exposure to EMFs.

The moral of this story is that mold and mold toxin removal must be done carefully, because heavy metal toxicity and EMF sensitivity can occur as a byproduct of mold removal. Mold, heavy metals, and electromagnetic fields work synergistically to damage the body, since the effects of each one compound and exacerbate the effects of the others. For this reason, I believe that these are three of the most dangerous toxins in our environment today, especially for those with chronic illness.

Water-Damaged Buildings and Chronic Inflammatory Response Syndrome

Note: The information for this section was taken by permission from Ritchie Shoemaker, MD, and the Mold Research Committee's July 2010 report, *Research Committee Report on Diagnosis and Treatment of Chronic Inflammatory Response Syndrome Caused by Exposure to the Interior Environment of Water-Damaged Buildings*.

The integrative and holistic medical community has typically focused upon mold and mold toxins (mycotoxins) as the sole causative agents of illness in susceptible people who have been exposed to water-damaged buildings. Yet some biotoxin experts, such as Ritchie Shoemaker, MD, author of *Mold Warriors* and the more recent *Surviving Mold*, have discovered that it isn't just mold that causes illness. According to Dr. Shoemaker, a variety of gram-negative bacteria, endotoxins, toxins made by a type of bacteria called actinomycetes and mycotoxins, as well as mold and other fungal species are all present in water-damaged buildings, and all cause disease. They individually and collectively manufacture toxins and activate inflammatory responses, which function synergistically to cause symptoms.

Furthermore, because people have differing immune responses to these pathogens and toxins, it is difficult to determine specifically which agents are causing what abnormal immune responses in the body, and how. It is also hard to determine which inflammatory processes are responsible for creating symptoms. What's more, inflammatory processes that are triggered by toxins and pathogens initiate a cascade of events in the body whereby other inflammatory processes get activated, so that it becomes difficult to determine which process was triggered by what other process or toxin.

The July 2010 *Research Committee Report on Diagnosis and Treatment of Chronic Inflammatory Response Syndrome Caused by Exposure to the Interior Environment of Water-Damaged Buildings* states that:

> "[According to the] US Government Accountability Office (GAO, 2008) report and the World Health Organization report (WHO, 2009), there are many compounds, both toxigens and inflamma-gens, present in the indoor air of a WDB (water-damaged building) that have been identified within the complex mixture found in the air and in the dust of the interior environments of WDB. Further, there is clear data showing that each of these compounds can initiate an inflammatory host response such that no single compound can be identified as the sole cause of the inflammatory responses seen in affected patients. Since many sources of inflammatory stimulus exist, some of which are synergistic, and no single causative agent within the WDB can be deemed to be solely responsible for the symptoms exhibited, the sole causative agent becomes the interior environment of the WDB itself."

Dr. Shoemaker and the other physicians and experts who compiled this report have named the condition that people suffer from following exposure to water-damaged buildings CIRS-WDB (Chronic Inflammatory Response Syndrome acquired following exposure to the interior environment of Water-Damaged Buildings). More than just mold toxicity, CIRS-WDB is multi-system, multi-symptom illness that can be effectively diagnosed and treated.

Diagnosis

Diagnosing CIRS-WDB involves: 1) identifying the patient's present and past exposure to water-damaged buildings; 2) performing a symptom analysis and identifying clusters of symptoms that have been found in others with the same illness, based on studies; 3) doing lab tests to identify unique groupings of biomarkers such as genetic markers, neuropeptides, inflammatory markers, and autoimmune processes that might indicate CIRS-WDB; and 4) doing a differential diagnosis, which involves comparing and contrasting the symptoms and clinical findings of similar diseases, to determine which one the patient is suffering from.

Symptoms

People with CIRS-WDB display a proven and consistent pattern of symptoms, although they have different immune responses to the cocktail of microbes and toxins found in water-damaged buildings. Common symptoms (some of which were mentioned earlier in this chapter) include: fatigue, weakness, aches, muscle cramps, unusual pain, ice-pick-like pain, headaches, light sensitivity, red eyes, blurred vision, tearing, sinus problems, cough, shortness of breath, abdominal pain, joint pain, diarrhea, morning stiffness, memory problems, focus/concentration problems, decreased ability to acquire new knowledge, word-recollection problems, confusion, disorientation, skin sensitivity, mood swings, sweats (especially night sweats), temperature-regulation problems, excessive thirst, increased urination, static shocks, numbness, tingling, vertigo, metallic taste in the mouth, and tremors.

Laboratory Tests

Lab tests can help to confirm the presence of CIRS-WDB, since the syndrome causes multiple immune marker abnormalities that can be detected through testing. These markers include: 1) abnormalities in the levels of regulatory neuropeptides melanocyte-stimulating hormone (MSH) and vasoactive intestinal polypeptide (VIP); 2) pro-inflammatory cytokines IL-1B, IL-6, 8, 12, and 13, as well as others; 3) split products of complement activation, especially C4a; 4) responses of hypoxia inducible factor, including, but not limited to, vascular endothelial growth factor (VEGF), erythropoietin, and transforming growth factor beta-1 (TGF B-1); and 5) cellular immunity. This type of cellular immunity includes effects on T-regulatory cells (Th-17 immunity impacting IL-17 and IL-23 functions) and auto-immunity—primarily antigliadin and anti-cardiolipin antibodies. Describing each of these laboratory markers and their role in CIRS-WDB is beyond the scope of this book; however, you can find a more in-depth description of each one at Dr. Shoemaker's website and in the above-mentioned report, which can be found at: http://www.survivingmold.com/legal-resources/publications/poa-position-statement-paper.

Some of these markers only measure the degree to which inflammation is present in the body. By themselves, they do not specifically indicate which types of toxins are causing inflammation, or how. They can help substantiate a diagnosis, however, when combined with a symptom analysis, an evaluation of potential exposure to water-damaged buildings, and other factors.

In addition to the lab tests, Dr. Shoemaker's visual contrast sensitivity (VCS) test can be taken online at www.survivingmold.com. This is another useful diagnostic tool that can help to confirm CIRS-WDB. Also, it is a good idea to test for the presence of certain immune response genes called HLA DR haplotypes, as these can indicate whether a person has a genetic defect which prevents them from being able to eliminate mold and other toxins implicated in CIRS-WDB.

Treatment

Studies indicate that the inflammatory processes triggered by exposure to water-damaged buildings don't abate by simply avoiding the place of exposure, or by remediating the affected structures. So even if a building is made "safe," the inflammation and toxins that result from exposure to toxic buildings will persist unless it is also treated and removed.

According to Dr. Shoemaker, only a series of specifically sequenced therapies can restore patients with CIRS-WDB back to health. Among other things, it's important to correct the series of abnormal immune and inflammatory responses in order for healing to occur. In the following section, I list the treatment components that Dr. Shoemaker has found to be essential when treating a CIRS-WDB patient. For more detailed information on these components and how to address them, as well as why each is important for healing from CIRS-WDB, see the above-mentioned report, which can also be found on Dr. Shoemaker's website: www.survivingmold.com.

Dr. Shoemaker's Protocol for Treating CIRS-WDB

Dr. Shoemaker's treatment regimen for CIRS-WDB is the result of thirteen years of work with over 6,000 patients. According to Dr. Shoemaker, all of the following steps are important for healing from CIRS-WDB, and should be undertaken in chronological order:

1. Remove the patient from exposure to water-damaged structures/buildings.

2. Orally administer cholestyramine or Welchol, to bind toxins, four times daily in therapeutic doses, until Visual Contrast Sensitivity (VCS) scores are normalized.

3. Eradicate commensal, biofilm-forming, multiply antibiotic-resistant coagulase negative staphylococci (bacteria).

4. Correct antigliadin antibody positivity (if present) by avoiding gluten for at least three months.

5. Normalize MMP-9 (an enzyme that delivers inflammatory elements to tissues).

6. Correct abnormal levels of antidiuretic hormone, as well as osmolality dysregulation (osmolality tests measure the concentration of all chemical particles found in the fluid part of the blood).

7. Correct androgen deficiencies (androgens are steroid hormones responsible for the development of male characteristics) and aromatase up-regulation (aromatase is an enzyme involved in the biosynthesis of estrogen hormones).

8. Correct abnormal C3a values. (C3a is an immune protein that aids in innate immunity).

9. Correct abnormal C4a values (the C4a test is one of the most commonly utilized and recognized lab markers of inflammation).

10. Correct elevated Transforming Growth Factor beta-1 (TGF β-1).

11. Replace Vasoactive Intestinal Peptide (VIP) if necessary (VIP regulates inflammation, among other things).

Treating Low MSH and MARCoNS

As noted on Dr. Shoemaker's website and in his books, one important indicator of mold toxicity (and biotoxin illness) is low levels of MSH, or melanocyte-stimulating hormone, which has multiple anti-inflammatory and neuro-hormonal regulatory functions. Nearly everyone with mold toxicity has low MSH levels. These levels can also be low in people with chronic Lyme disease and in those who have a type of chronic sinus infection called "multiply antibiotic-resistant coagulase negative staphylococci" (MARCoNS). People with mold toxicity may not recover until this infection is treated, so it may be important to discover whether the infection is playing a role in disease. Doing an Api-Staph culture is one way to diagnose MARCoNS. Treating the sinus cavities by mixing in a neti pot one-half teaspoon of sea salt, xylitol, and baking soda is one effective way to treat this infection. Staph infections in the nose upset the hypothalamus and affect hormone production. It is important to treat them for this reason.

If you suspect that you have mold toxicity and/or CIRS-WDB, you'll want to learn as much as possible about it in order to put together an effective treatment regimen and to avoid re-exposure. Some good resources for this purpose include Dr. Schaller's book, *Mold Illness and Mold Remediation Made Simple: Removing Mold Toxins From Bodies and Sick Buildings*; Dr. Shoemaker's books and website, www.survivingmold. com (which includes the above-mentioned report), and Richard Loyd's website, www.royalrife.com.

Chapter Five

Pyroluria/Heavy Metal Toxicity

Many people with Lyme disease—up to 80 percent, by some estimates—suffer from a condition called pyroluria, also known among the medical community as kryptopyrroluria (KPU) or hemopyrrollactamuria (HPU). This is a condition in which the body doesn't effectively synthesize heme to make hemoglobin (which is used to carry iron in red blood cells), and instead produces a useless by-product of heme, sometimes referred to as the "mauve factor" which is excreted by the body. As it is eliminated, it binds with certain nutrients, especially minerals, and causes severe deficiencies of these nutrients in the body, as well as heavy metal toxicity.

Pyroluria was first discovered by Abram Hoffer, MD, PhD, in 1958, in conjunction with C. C. Pfeiffer, MD, PhD. They found that the mauve substance would bind and deactivate the essential nutrients pyridoxine (B-6) and zinc in the body, and that schizophrenics had high amounts of the substance in their urine. These doctors, along with other researchers, then tested thousands of patients in several different mental hospitals for the presence of the mauve substance. Their findings are summarized in an article that Dr. Hoffer wrote, which was published in 1995 in *The Journal of Orthomolecular Medicine*:

> "It [the mauve factor] was present mostly in schizophrenic patients but was also present in one-quarter of other non-schizophrenic patients including depressions, alcoholics, anxiety states, and in children with learning and behavioral disorders. It was rarely present in normal subjects, and was present in ten percent of a non-psychiatric

stressed population drawn from the surgical wards of the hospital. To my surprise, it was found in most cases of lung cancer."

Drs. Hoffer and Pfeiffer later named the mauve substance "kryptopyrrole," and Dr. Pfeiffer named the disease that it caused "pyrolleuria," now more commonly known as pyroluria.

Subsequent discoveries have revealed that in addition to zinc and vitamin B-6, people with pyroluria are often also deficient in biotin, manganese, molybdenum, chromium, and other trace elements. These deficiencies create dysfunctional biochemical processes and debilitate the immune system, resulting in both psychological and physical symptoms.

While Lyme disease may cause pyroluria, it can also be inherited or triggered by childhood trauma. When inherited, pyroluria may create a predisposition to Lyme disease by depleting nutrients from the body and causing immune dysfunction. The person becomes then susceptible to illness from tick-borne infections. As with other causes of disease mentioned in this book, it's difficult to know which came first—illness from tick-borne infections or illness from the pyroluria and accompanying immune system weakness. Yet it is important to treat both conditions, as both are major contributing factors to chronic illness.

Pyroluria is prevalent in people who have other illnesses besides Lyme disease. According to the Direct Health Care Access II Laboratory (http://kryptopyrrole.com), clinical trials have revealed that elevated pyrrole levels exist in over 70 percent of people who suffer from depression and schizophrenia (Hoffer); in 50 percent of those with autism, and in 30 percent of those with ADD or ADHD. It is also common in people who have high levels of heavy metal toxicity.

Pyroluria causes psychiatric symptoms such as anxiety and irritability, and plays a role in other mental disorders. When it is the primary cause of these disorders, treating it can bring about a complete resolution of, or significant reduction in symptoms. Symptoms of pyroluria and Lyme disease, particularly the psychiatric ones, overlap. It can be difficult to discern whether the symptoms that are present in a person who has both conditions are caused primarily by pyroluria or by Lyme. For this reason, it is important for people with Lyme disease to get tested for pyroluria, because if the condition is present, treating it may be necessary for a full recovery. Pyroluria suppresses the immune system by creating severe deficiencies of minerals that the body needs to fight disease, especially zinc (which plays a major role in immune function), and can lead to symptoms similar to those found in chronic Lyme disease. It also creates heavy metal toxicity, which further weakens immune function and precludes healing.

Thus, testing for and treating pyroluria shouldn't be considered optional for people with chronic Lyme disease, or for people with illnesses that mimic Lyme, such as fibromyalgia and chronic fatigue syndrome. A few Lyme disease sufferers I have spoken with have told me that treating pyroluria has produced greater improvements to their overall well-being than any other treatment that they have done. For these people, pyroluria may have been a more significant cause of disease than tick-borne infections, which are almost always considered by practitioners and patients alike to be the most important cause of symptoms.

Pyroluria Symptoms

According to the Direct Health Care Access II Laboratory, Inc., which tests for kryptopyrroles:

> "... symptoms of excess urinary kryptopyrrole first manifest themselves as behavioral abnormalities. Although children tend to be more easily diagnosed than adults, the symptoms are consistent: poor tolerance of physical and emotional stress, mood swings, depression, (and) sensitivity to light, noise and other tactile sensitivities. Later, symptoms can range from severe depression to chronic schizophrenia. Accompanying physical symptoms can include pain, seizures, even complete physical debilitation."

Other symptoms of pyroluria include:

- Poor dream recall
- White spots on the fingernails
- Menstrual cycle irregularities
- Sexual dysfunction
- Insomnia

- Hypoglycemia
- Tremors, shaking, spasms
- Environmental and food allergies
- Poor morning appetite
- Cold hands and feet
- Anxiety/withdrawal
- Paranoia/hallucinations
- Knee and joint pain
- Attention deficits
- Anemia that responds to B-6 supplementation
- Retention of toxic metals and environmental toxins
- Abdominal tenderness
- Course eyebrows
- Constipation
- Rage, irritability
- Memory and cognitive problems
- Skin that burns easily

Not all of these symptoms are present in everyone with pyroluria. As with other conditions, the symptom presentation varies from person to person. Psychiatric symptoms most strongly indicate the condition, especially when kryptopyrrole levels are exceptionally high.

Testing for Pyroluria

Pyroluria is diagnosed clinically, by doing a symptom analysis, along with a urine test, which measures kryptopyrrole levels. The urine test can be done through labs such as Natural Health Innovations, Inc. (www.naturalhealthinnovations.net) and Direct Health Care Access II Laboratory (www.kryptopyrrole.com). Other labs may test for kryptopyrroles, as well. To get the most accurate lab test results, it's important to avoid all supplements, especially those containing zinc, biotin, and vitamin B-6, for five to seven days prior to collecting a urine sample. Some doctors suggest that their patients do a 24-hour urine collection instead of a single morning collection, since the release of kryptopyrroles from the body is sporadic and may not be present in a single urine collection.

Some people test negative for pyroluria, although they have the condition. If symptoms indicate pyroluria, doing an empirical trial of a pyroluria treatment protocol can help to confirm a diagnosis. This involves replenishing the nutrients that are missing from the body by taking therapeutic doses of them.

Other Laboratory Results That Indicate Pyroluria

Other lab tests may be useful for confirming a pyroluria diagnosis, especially when kryptopyrrol test results are negative. Below are additional lab test indicators that may help to establish a diagnosis:

- White blood cell counts of less than 5,000/mcL (caused by low levels of zinc).
- High copper levels, low serum zinc levels, or a poor zinc-to-copper ratio. (Zinc and copper compete for absorption in the body, and can therefore displace one another).
- Poor methylation. Through his research, Dr. Hoffer learned that symptoms of pyroluria can be muted in people who under-methylate (as well as in those with obsessive-compulsive disorder. Methylation is explained in Chapter Eight).

Why Pyroluria Treatment Causes Symptoms of Heavy Metal Toxicity

People who have both Lyme disease and pyroluria tend to feel worse during the initial phases of pyroluria treatment, which involves nutrient replacement therapy. Based on anecdotal reports of those who have undergone treatment, the "feeling worse" stage may last anywhere from several months up to a year or more. This happens because people with Lyme disease and pyroluria tend to have high levels of heavy metal toxicity. Heavy metals occupy the same receptor sites on cells as minerals. When the body is given high replacement doses of minerals, it begins to displace heavy metals from the cells. This causes a profound detoxification reaction that can continue on and off for months. The reaction is prolonged because it takes time for the body to replenish its mineral stores and displace metals, especially when mineral deficiencies are severe. People with severe mineral deficiencies also tend to have high levels of heavy metals in their bodies. It can take time to remove all of these. Once the cellular receptor sites become mostly occupied by minerals, the body ceases to release metals and there are fewer places for the metals to latch onto. Heavy metal toxicity is another major contributing factor to chronic illness, so treating pyroluria as part of a comprehensive heavy metal detoxification protocol, can help to more effectively remove metals from the body.

Regardless of whether the body has high or low amounts of heavy metal toxins, the metals that damage it the most are those that occupy mineral receptor sites on cells. The minerals that should normally occupy these sites are of critical biological importance. Displacing any heavy metals from these sites and replacing them with essential minerals is therefore crucial for healing.

When heavy metals are displaced from cellular receptor sites by pyroluria treatment, they can cause more severe detoxification reactions in the body than what would normally occur as a result of heavy metal treatments. The detoxification process is healthy, because it replaces toxic heavy metals with minerals that the body needs, but can also be dangerous if not handled properly. When toxic heavy metals are displaced from the cells into systemic circulation, they can build up in the blood to toxic levels—much faster than the kidneys, liver, and lymphatic system can eliminate them. Any metals the body cannot eliminate will then get redistributed throughout the body, where they can cause further, even irreversible, damage to the organs and tissues. To prevent this from happening, it is essential for people with pyroluria to work with a healthcare practitioner who is experienced not only in treating pyroluria, but also heavy metal toxicity.

Once the cellular receptor sites become mostly occupied by minerals, the body ceases to release toxic metals, resulting in fewer sites to which these toxins can bind. It is vital to support the body during the heavy metal detoxification process that accompanies pyroluria treatment. The topic of heavy metal detoxification will be addressed in greater detail at the end of this chapter.

Nutrient Deficiencies and Symptoms Caused by Pyroluria

Pyroluria causes nutrient deficiencies, which can result in a multitude of problems in the body, including immune and neurological dysfunction. Specific symptoms that can result from each of the nutrient deficiencies caused by pyroluria are described in the following paragraphs.

Zinc

Zinc plays a powerful role in neurotransmitter synthesis. Since neurotransmitters regulate mood and cognitive function, deficiencies can cause depression and other mental disorders. Zinc is also strongly involved in immune function, including white blood cell production, so people with low levels of this mineral often have low white blood cell counts. This, in turn, makes the body more susceptible to infections and toxins.

Deficiencies also result in delayed wound healing, and can cause low stomach acid, diminished collagen levels, macular degeneration, dandruff, hyperactivity, loss of appetite, and bone loss. Because zinc is an antioxidant, lowered levels also lead to oxidative stress and inflammation.

Vitamin B-6 (Pyridoxine)

Vitamin B-6 deficiencies are thought to be rare among the general population; however, in those with pyroluria, they are common. B-6 deficiencies can cause insomnia, irritability, depression, cognitive dysfunction, muscle weakness, poor nutrient absorption, and anemia. Because of B-6's important role in serotonin synthesis, insufficient levels of this vitamin lead to neurotransmitter deficiencies, and to neurological problems such as depression. A lack of B-6 can also cause poor dream recall.

Biotin

Biotin deficiency, which is also found in those with pyroluria, can cause rashes, dry skin, fine or brittle hair, hair loss, conjunctivitis, dermatitis, muscle pain, and neurological symptoms such as depression, lethargy, and numbness and tingling of the extremities. Biotin is necessary for cell growth, fatty acid synthesis, and fat and amino acid metabolism. Deficiencies result in inefficient metabolic processes. Biotin deficiency is also associated with many aspects of the aging process.

Manganese

Deficiencies of manganese have been linked to ataxia (poor gait), dermatitis, weak tendons and ligaments, hearing loss, joint pain, inflammation, and arthritis. Deficiencies may also cause or contribute to the development of diabetes, Parkinson's disease, osteoporosis, and epilepsy, because manganese is essential for normal growth, glucose utilization, lipid (fat) metabolism, and thyroid hormone production. Because manganese interferes with iron absorption, people with pyroluria who also have iron deficiencies (including most women with Lyme disease), may also want to supplement with a food-based iron product while on a pyroluria protocol that involves taking manganese. The iron should not be taken at the same time as the manganese.

Molybdenum

Molybdenum is most highly concentrated in the liver and kidneys. It plays an essential role in detoxification, so deficiencies can disrupt or cause detoxification processes to be inefficient. Molybdenum deficiency is indicated by liver dysfunction, and symptoms such as jaundice, nausea, and fatigue. Because the liver is constantly stressed in chronically ill people, it may be difficult to identify this deficiency through a symptom analysis alone. Moderate deficiencies of molybdenum result in sulfite toxicity, which can cause headaches, tachycardia, vomiting, and nausea. Molybdenum also helps the body utilize energy from fats and carbohydrates; deficiencies of this mineral may cause fatigue. Molybdenum also plays a role in iron utilization, tooth decay prevention, and in maintaining fertility, mental clarity, and blood sugar balance.

Most of the aforementioned nutrients play an important role in neurological and immune function, detoxification, and blood sugar balance. Correcting for deficiencies of these nutrients may help to heal the body of a multitude of symptoms, some of which may be mistakenly assumed to be due to tick-borne infections.

Pyroluria Treatment

Treating pyroluria involves taking relatively high doses of some, or all, of the aforementioned nutrients, to replace deficiencies in the body. Nutrient replacement therapy must sometimes be done for life, depending upon the cause of pyroluria. Eliminating microbes, in some cases, may enable the body to correct the processes that caused pyroluria in the first place, thus eliminating the need for lifelong therapy. Because people with pyroluria have varying degrees of vitamin and mineral deficiencies, replacement doses of nutrients must be based on lab test results, or the results of other diagnostic testing methods such as applied kinesiology or bioenergetic testing (the latter of which are described in other chapters of this book). To avoid overdosing on nutrients, people with pyroluria should have their mineral levels monitored periodically by a healthcare practitioner, especially during the initial months of treatment.

The required nutrient doses will decrease over time as the body begins to build up its nutrient reserves. Once it has built up sufficient reserves, maintenance doses of the nutrients should be taken, usually for life. Maintenance doses may be half of the initial therapeutic doses, but again, it depends upon each person's biochemistry.

Recommended Nutrient Doses

(Warning: The following nutrient dosages and recommendations are, in some cases, much higher than what is recommended by the FDA. Anyone who is considering taking high doses of any of these minerals should first consult a licensed health care practitioner and get tested, to determine whether and how much of each nutrient they need. Several of the nutrients described in the following sections can be toxic at high doses and create potentially life-threatening reactions when taken in excess of the body's needs).

Zinc. Therapeutic doses of zinc may range from 20–80 mg of elemental zinc, based on anecdotal reports from those who have treated pyroluria.

Maintenance doses may be 10–40 mg. Because zinc is measured according to the form in which it is processed, it is important to discover whether zinc supplement labels reflect the elemental form or not.

Confusion over zinc supplement labeling has led at least one person with Lyme disease to severely overdose on zinc, and suffer from life-threatening symptoms. Furthermore, excessive zinc intake can result in severe copper deficiencies, which can also produce life-threatening symptoms. Information on how to prevent copper deficiencies will be described later in this chapter. It is vital to test the body's zinc levels before taking any amount of zinc which exceeds the FDA's recommended daily allowances.

Some people may experience nausea when they first start taking zinc, which may be a sign of hypochlorhydria, or low stomach acid. This tends to resolve over time. Taking zinc with food may also alleviate this symptom.

Manganese. Hypothetically, and based upon anecdotal reports, the amount of manganese that should be taken during pyroluria treatment ranges from 7–15 mg per day. Again, it's best to measure how much the body needs, rather than relying upon a general guideline or one doctor's specific protocol.

B-6. Vitamin B-6 doses may range from 75–150 mg per day (on average). Most people do best by taking a combination of both B-6 and pyridoxal phosphate, (P5P), which is a more bioavailable form of B-6.

These guidelines are meant to provide a general idea of the replacement doses that are generally needed to treat pyroluria in the initial therapeutic stages of treatment (which may last for several months or more). All of the nutrients that are described in this chapter should be included in a core treatment protocol for pyroluria, unless test results and symptoms indicate otherwise.

BioPure (www.biopureus.com) has formulated a product called CORE, which contains all of the replacement minerals and vitamins required to reverse the deficiencies caused by pyroluria. This may be a convenient product for those who don't wish to take all of their nutrients separately.

Not everyone reacts positively to the CORE product, however. While the reasons for this are unknown, it may be that some people need different doses of some of the nutrients contained within the CORE product, or that their bodies are only able to process the nutrients in a different form. It may be more beneficial for some people to take the nutrients separately. Doing this also allows for more control over the dosing of each nutrient and for the ability to take the nutrients in differing ratios.

For others, taking the CORE product may be an effective and convenient way to replace most of the nutrients that their bodies are missing. Therapeutic doses of the CORE product can range from 4–8 capsules per day (based on user reports). Maintenance doses are usually about half of that. That said, sensitive or severely mercury-toxic people may only be able to tolerate one or two capsules at the outset of treatment, as higher doses may displace excessive amounts of heavy metals that their bodies aren't equipped to remove.

Considerations in Pyroluria Treatment

The amount and type of each nutrient that people with pyroluria need or can tolerate, especially in the initial phases of treatment, depends upon many factors, in addition to the body's current nutritional status or degree of heavy metal toxicity.

Other factors that should be considered when deciding upon a pyroluria treatment regimen and corresponding heavy metal detoxification protocol include: 1) the strength of the immune system, especially adrenal gland function; 2) co-morbid conditions that are being concurrently treated, such as Lyme disease; 3) the level of heavy metal toxicity in the body; 4) the level and type of nutrient deficiencies present; 4) the body's ability to detoxify; and 5) the person's emotional well-being and amount of emotional support available. A pyroluria protocol can initially exacerbate depression and psychiatric symptoms due to the release of metals.

Evaluating all of these factors is critical before starting pyroluria treatment. The body may require high doses of certain minerals to replace those that are missing, but it may not initially tolerate high amounts of such minerals (and other nutrients), for the reasons I just described. This means that it may take some people longer than others to reap the benefits of pyroluria treatment.

Before deciding upon how much of each nutrient to take, it may also be a good idea to collectively evaluate all of the supplements that you are currently taking. Taking too many supplements can stress the body, because even though it may require fifty different substances to correct for multiple infections, toxins, and nutrient deficiencies, the body can process only so many of these substances at once. Any supplement that the body is unable to use, it processes as a toxin, which requires valuable energy. While the body may require many things to heal, it's not always prudent (nor cost-effective nor convenient) to take fifty different supplements daily. Sometimes better results may be achieved by taking ten well-chosen remedies before moving on to others. Pushing the body to do too much can result in treatment setbacks. Combining treatments is a delicate balancing act. Certain problems won't be resolved unless others are also, yet it is possible to impose too much work upon the body by giving it too many supplements or treatments at once.

The Importance of Replacing Copper and Iron during Pyroluria Treatment

Zinc, manganese, and vitamin B-6 all deplete copper in the body. Copper levels should be periodically measured during pyroluria treatment. This can be done through a red blood cell mineral test. The need for copper replacement can also be evaluated using applied kinesiology (muscle testing) or EAV/EDS-type biofeedback devices. (These are described more in-depth in Chapter Six). After several months of taking high levels of zinc, manganese, and vitamin B-6 (all of which are copper antagonists), it usually becomes necessary to continually supply the body with 2–6 mg of copper daily. Copper also plays an important role in helping the body to fight disease. Severe copper deficiencies are life-threatening and have been reported as a result of excess zinc supplementation; thus, it is important to continually monitor the body's level of this mineral.

It is also important to monitor iron levels during pyroluria treatment, and supplement for deficiencies as necessary. High levels of copper, manganese, or zinc can result in iron depletion. It is very important to keep all of these minerals in balance, since they have antagonistic effects upon one another. For example, high levels of zinc can result in low levels of both copper and iron. Similarly, high levels of copper can result in low levels of zinc and iron. For this reason, iron, copper, and zinc should be taken at separate intervals throughout the day, and their levels in the body continually monitored.

Some people with chronic illness and Lyme disease suffer from hemochromatosis, a potentially dangerous genetic condition that results from having excessively high levels of iron in the body. Such people obviously do not require iron supplementation, because their iron levels are already too high.

Heavy Metal Detoxification

Because pyroluria treatment displaces heavy metals, it's important to concurrently detoxify the body of heavy metals while taking high doses of minerals. Healthcare practitioners who treat pyroluria should not only thoroughly understand pyroluria and Lyme disease, but also heavy metal chelation. Heavy metal removal can be difficult and dangerous. Mistakes in treatment can cause displaced metals to cause irreversible harm and further damage to the tissues and organs as the metals find and bind to new receptor sites in the body. Practitioners need to know how to effectively bind and eliminate the metals that get released during treatment.

Regardless of whether a person has pyroluria, removing heavy metals from the body is important for healing from chronic illnesses of all kinds. Heavy metal toxicity is another major cause of symptoms in people with Lyme disease. Many Lyme-literate doctors recommend removing heavy metals from the body for a full recovery. It can be said that almost everyone, if not everyone, has some level of heavy metal toxicity due to the plethora of metal toxins in the air, water, and food supply; however, people with Lyme disease and chronic illness are particularly susceptible to the effects of toxins because their bodies' ability to detoxify is usually compromised by infections. Also, some researchers believe that tick-borne pathogens may preferentially store metal toxins in the body, in a strategic attempt to use them in ways that would enable their survival and compromise the immune system. People with tick-borne illness often cannot eliminate heavy metals and other environmental toxins as easily as people who are not infected with tick-borne pathogens. Their bodies contain higher amounts of these toxins as a result.

Fortunately, by treating pyroluria, this other major cause of illness in people with Lyme disease and chronic illness gets effectively addressed, as well. It, in effect, "kills two birds with one stone," since it not only restores the body's immune, neurological, and other functions by replenishing the body with essential nutrients, but also eliminates heavy metals, one of the most immune-suppressive types of toxins in our environment today.

While many substances are purported to be useful for chelating, binding, and removing metals from the tissues and organs, controversy exists over the best way to effectively and safely do this. Chelators mobilize metals from stored places throughout the body and bring them out of the tissues and into the bloodstream. Binders attach to the circulating metals and help the body to excrete them. They do this partially by preventing them from being reabsorbed by bile (and then re-circulated throughout the body) once they reach the gastrointestinal tract.

Chlorella and cilantro are two popular natural remedies used by some people for heavy metal removal. Both substances mobilize metals from their receptor sites, although cilantro is better at mobilizing mercury in the brain. Chlorella both mobilizes and binds metals. Some heavy metal chelation experts, however, such as Andrew Cutler, PhD, PE, who is also author of the book, *Amalgam Illness: Diagnosis and Treatment*, believe chlorella and cilantro to be weak chelators and binders of metals and therefore, potentially dangerous. When a heavy metal chelator forms weak bonds with a heavy metal, it creates the potential for that heavy metal to be dropped by the binder on its way out of the body, and redistributed to other organs, where it can cause further damage.

According to Dr. Cutler, Dimercaptosuccinic acid (DMSA) and/or Dimercaptopropanesulfonic acid (DMPS), along with alpha-lipoic acid, are a safer and more effective combination for heavy metal chelation and removal than chlorella and other natural substances. He also contends that there are very specific guidelines for the use of these substances, including how and when to dose them. As previously mentioned, the body's ability to detoxify, its overall toxic burden, and other factors must be taken into account when formulating a treatment plan. Dr. Cutler has developed protocols and guidelines for heavy metal chelation. These should not be casually implemented without thoroughly understanding his entire approach to chelation. They should also be administered under the guidance of a healthcare practitioner who thoroughly understands heavy metal chelation.

Cardiologist James Roberts, MD, FACC, a board-certified chelation expert and co-author with Stephen Sinatra, MD, of *Reverse Heart Disease Now*, advocates DMSA and DMPS as well as EDTA for heavy metal chelation. More information on how he uses these substances can be found on his website: www.heartfixer.com. According to Dr. Roberts, DMSA and DMPS are more effective for removing mercury from the body, while EDTA is more effective for removing lead. He notes on his website that DMPS is a stronger chelating agent than DMSA, but that DMSA is more effective for removing mercury located in the neurological system. He contends that EDTA is relatively ineffective when administered orally, but when used intravenously, is very effective. He also believes that oral zeolite may be somewhat beneficial for removing metals (although its effects are not as powerful as those of the former agents), and that glutathione is useful for helping the body to bind mercury so that the body can more effectively eliminate it.

As with Dr. Cutler's protocols, however, it is best to thoroughly study Dr. Roberts' approach before attempting treatment. Do not formulate a chelation protocol based upon a few recommendations from his website or any other source, including this book. These sources are only intended to provide a broad overview of heavy metal chelation and the agents that are used for heavy metal removal.

While widely recommended among those who understand heavy metal chelation best, DMSA and DMPS may not be safe to take on a daily basis over a period of many months. Unfortunately, during pyroluria treatment, the body may be releasing heavy metals for a year or more. The person undergoing treatment will require toxin binders for as long as this is happening. Taking intermittent breaks from pyroluria treatment, or rotating DMSA and DMPS with other chelating/binding agents, may be a good idea, even though these other binding agents may not have been proven in studies to be as strong or effective as DMSA/DMPS. For some people, though, they may be a viable option. Examples of alternative heavy metal binding substances include: microsilica, chlorella, glutathione, and zeolite. Microsilica is thought to be especially helpful for binding metals in the gut and for encouraging the movement of other metals toward the gut.

During the therapeutic stages of my own pyroluria treatment, I rotated DMSA and alpha-lipoic acid with microsilica and chlorella, which my doctor determined to be the best regimen for me, based on applied kinesiology test results. What was beneficial for me may not work for another person, however. It's important to work with a doctor who doesn't make treatment decisions based on popular or fad protocols, but instead upon scientific research, clinical experience, and the patient's individual biochemistry.

Also, chelators and binders may function differently in how they remove metals from the body. For instance, cilantro, an herb from the parsley family, mobilizes mercury from the brain, but it doesn't create an adequately strong bond with the heavy metal to usher it out of the body. Therefore, it is important to take it in combination with a binder such as DMSA and/or alpha-lipoic acid. Chlorella binds metals, but may not mobilize metals from the brain. It must be used in conjunction with a substance that crosses the blood-brain barrier, such as alpha-lipoic acid.

In Summary

Treating pyroluria may resolve symptoms that were initially attributed solely to tick-borne infections. Pyroluria may be just as an important cause of symptoms as Lyme disease, especially when symptoms are strongly neurological. Pyroluria depletes essential nutrients from the body, especially zinc and vitamin B-6, and thereby hampers immune function, making recovery from tick-borne and other conditions difficult. Pyroluria should be treated whenever it is present in chronic illness, as it is sometimes a major cause of immune dysfunction and symptoms. It can also be what allows tick-borne and other infections to establish a foothold in the body.

Treatment for pyroluria must be undertaken with utmost care, as inappropriate nutrient dosages and improper heavy metal removal protocols can severely damage the body. Taking higher doses of nutrients than are called for by the U.S. RDA (recommended dietary allowance) guidelines can be risky and dangerous if the body doesn't need those nutrients. Pyroluria treatment is also experimental, and there is no such thing as a "one size fits all" protocol. Treatments should be undertaken only under the guidance and supervision of a competent physician who thoroughly understands both pyroluria and heavy metal removal.

Chapter Six

Parasites

Lyme-literate practitioners are increasingly finding that parasites are a major cause of symptoms and illness in their patients with Lyme disease. Unfortunately, parasites are often treated as an ancillary or secondary problem to tick-borne infections—as a nuisance to the immune system, but not the real reason why symptoms are present.

If the body has parasites, it's sometimes because the immune system has been weakened by other factors, such as tick-borne infections, but parasites also play a main role in immune suppression and illness. And to assume that parasites can be effectively treated by simply taking a couple of anti-parasitic remedies such as wormwood or Alinia for a couple of weeks is to underestimate their tenacity and importance in the overall symptom picture.

Lyme-literate doctors usually treat their chronically ill Lyme patients for many months or years with multiple antibiotics and herbs. Good doctors regularly rotate their patients' regimens to ensure that the infections are thoroughly and adequately treated. But what if symptoms of Lyme disease are present and the tick-borne infections are difficult to eradicate because parasites are also keeping the immune system in a weakened state? What if parasites are a bigger problem for the body than tick-borne infections? At the 2011 Conference "A Deep Look Beyond Lyme," Simon Yu, MD, presented numerous case studies that demonstrated how his chronically ill patients, who were initially diagnosed with conditions from autism to cancer, Lyme disease, and MS, would improve radically after parasite treatment. They also responded better to nutritional treatments after their parasites were eliminated. Dr. Yu contends that if you can rid the body of parasites, sometimes symptoms of other infections will automatically resolve. He believes that parasite treatment can be effective for healing chronic illness when all other treatments fail.

Dr. Yu has also found that, as with Lyme disease and MS, parasites cause lesions on the brain and other Lyme-like symptoms. These symptoms are often blamed on tick-borne infections. Based on the opinions and experience of Dr. Yu, it seems worthwhile for people with Lyme disease to investigate the possibility that their symptoms are being caused, at least in part, by parasitic infections.

Another well-respected Lyme-literate doctor whom I interviewed (whose name I must withhold for privacy) contends that some people who believe that Lyme organisms are their main problem are really suffering from multiple parasitic infections. He believes that if patients are treated for parasites first, then they may only need antibiotic therapy for their tick-borne infections for weeks or months, instead of years.

Additionally, many people with Lyme disease suffer from psychiatric symptoms, which are usually attributed to tick-borne infections, but studies have shown that psychiatric symptoms may also be caused by parasites. For instance, an abstract of a 1997 article that was published in *Psychological Bulletin* states: "The title of a 1930s article asked the question, 'Stupidity or Hookworm?' In this article, the authors discuss research that attempts to answer the question of whether intestinal worms; namely, hookworm, whipworm, and roundworm, harm the mental performance of their hosts. After introducing the biology and epidemiology of intestinal worms, the authors present the historical background to the problem. They review research from the 1910s through the 1990s; (and conclude) there is evidence that high intensities of worms can affect mental performance . . ."

Ascertaining the role and importance of parasites in chronic illness is difficult. As with so many other types of pathogens, lab tests fail to detect many types of parasites. Parasites can also affect nearly every organ and system in the body, and therefore produce symptoms that overlap with those of Lyme disease. There is a also the mistaken assumption among some people in the medical community that parasites exist only in third-world countries, and that if people happen to have them, they are more treatable than tick-borne infections. But parasites are just as prevalent in developed nations as in developing nations. Some experts, such as Mehmet C. Oz, MD, believe that over 90 percent of the population of the United States is infected with parasites. International travel has also brought many types of parasites into the developed world that initially only existed in developing nations.

Another reason why parasites are often ignored in people with Lyme disease is because there is an outdated mentality among some practitioners in the Lyme disease community that if the tick-borne infections are effectively treated, then the immune system will take care of the other infections and problems in the body on its own. This is a mistaken assumption. Parasites can be much more tenacious and adaptable to the body than bacteria such as *Borrelia*. They can be more resistant to the body's defenses and antimicrobial remedies than bacterial tick-borne pathogens. If intelligent, prolonged, and aggressive treatment regimens are necessary for eradicating tick-borne pathogens, then how much more aggressive should treatment for parasites be, taking into account their incredible ability to survive in a hostile environment?

Parasites don't just suppress the immune system, deplete the body of nutrients, and cause symptoms. They also harbor other pathogens and toxins, including tick-borne microbes and viruses. Therefore, treating the body for bacteria, viruses and environmental toxins may not be completely effective unless parasites are also treated. Until the parasites are killed, it may be impossible to eliminate these other pathogens and toxins.

Unfortunately, as with tick-borne infections, not enough research has been conducted on effective parasite treatments for humans. This is partly because the medical community has not yet identified many types of parasites that infect humans. Also, many parasites cannot be tested for via conventional labs, so effective treatments can't be developed for them.

Fortunately, increasing numbers of holistic doctors are finding parasites in their patients with Lyme disease when they use unconventional testing methods to detect them. (More about such methods will be described subsequently). People with tick-borne infections tend to have higher numbers of parasites than the general population. This may be due to the fact that tick-borne infections suppress immune function, or because the immune system was dysfunctional to begin with. When immune function is weak, the body becomes susceptible to disease from all kinds of pathogens, including tick-borne infections and parasites.

(Note: In the Appendix of this book, I note some of the latest antimicrobial treatments for *Borrelia, Babesia, Bartonella,* and other important tick-borne infections. I have put these in the Appendix because the focus of this book is on other major causes of illness in people with Lyme, besides tick-borne infections. Also many other good books have already been written that focus on treatment for these infections. In this book, I discuss mostly mold and parasites, because I believe that these are often overlooked as major causes of disease in people with Lyme, and that they can be a primary, or more important, cause of symptoms than tick-borne infections. While I realize that *Babesia* is a tick-borne parasitic organism, for the purposes of this chapter, I will be discussing parasites that aren't commonly identified or recognized in people with tick-borne infections, and which aren't typically transmitted along with *Borrelia*).

Types of Parasites

Many types of parasites cause infection in humans, and some are more virulent and damaging to the body than others. Protozoa comprise the majority of parasites. These microscopic organisms are invisible to the naked eye. They can cause great damage to the body as they multiply and invade the organs and tissues. Amoebas, giardia, blastocystis hominis, plasmodium, and toxoplasma are examples of protozoa. Among the larger types of parasites are nematodes (such as roundworms, pinworms, filaria, and hookworms) and trematoda, which are flatworms (including flukes and tapeworms).

Parasites enter the body through the mouth or skin, and are principally transmitted through water (tap water as well as lakes, ponds, and streams), contaminated or uncooked food, soil, pets, sexual contact, and fecal matter.

From their point of entry in the body, parasites then migrate and reproduce in different organs and tissues. This is why they can produce a variety of symptoms, which aren't limited to the gastrointestinal tract, although the GI tract (both the large and small intestines) is the preferred colonization site for many. Other preferred sites of colonization include the brain, liver, lungs, and muscles, as well as the heart. Because parasites don't just colonize the digestive tract but also other parts of the body, they can do great damage to the body.

Symptoms of Parasitic Infection

Discerning parasites via a symptom analysis alone can be difficult. As with the other conditions described in this book, symptoms of parasitic infection overlap with those of other infections and problems. Combining a symptom analysis with test results, and doing an empirical treatment trial, may be the best strategy for determining whether parasites are active and causing symptoms.

Parasites can be the entire or partial cause of chronic fatigue syndrome, fibromyalgia, hypoglycemia, depression, and other chronic health conditions, especially those that involve the GI tract such as food allergies, irritable bowel syndrome, Crohn's disease, and colitis.

Ann Louise Gittleman, MS, CNS, in her well-researched book on parasites, *Guess What Came To Dinner?* writes: "The following are warning signs for parasites: constipation, diarrhea, gas and bloating, irritable bowel syndrome, joint and muscle aches and pains, anemia, allergy, skin conditions, granulomas, nervousness, sleep disturbances, teeth grinding, chronic fatigue, and immune dysfunction."

All of these symptoms are also found in people with tick-borne infections. It may be no surprise that parasites are so easily and commonly overlooked by Lyme-literate doctors. While these symptoms are among the most important indicators of parasitic infection, this list isn't all-inclusive of the symptoms that can occur in people with parasites.

Simon Yu, MD, in his book, *Accidental Cure*, has compiled a list of additional symptoms that are found in people with parasitic infections. He compares these to symptoms that are found in people with allergies. He writes: "Many symptoms that indicate a parasite infection also indicate allergy problems and vice-versa." Such symptoms include brain fog, fatigue, bloating and other GI disturbances, weight changes, immune deficiency, and ulcerative colitis.

Testing for Parasites

Conventional labs look for parasites via a stool analysis, but fail to detect them for many reasons. First, as previously mentioned, many parasites exist outside of the gastrointestinal (GI) tract, in other parts of the body. It is therefore impossible to obtain them from a stool sample. Second, stool tests, even those from reputable labs, fail to detect many types of parasites in the GI tract. This happens for many reasons, including the fact that many types of parasites don't appear in random stool samples. Some adhere strongly to GI tract tissue and are not excreted by the body. Taking several stool samples may produce better outcomes for certain types of parasites. Even then, some infections may be missed. Third, lab tests haven't yet been developed for many types of parasites that reside in humans. Even if people test positive for one or two types of parasites via a stool simple, there may yet be five or ten other types of parasites in their bodies that lab tests will fail to detect.

Because of these factors, it's important to use unconventional testing methods to diagnose parasitic infections, in addition to a symptom-based, or clinical, diagnosis. For instance, applied kinesiology techniques (e.g., muscle testing) can be effective for detecting parasites if the practitioner is proficient in the techniques and has the necessary tools to test for many different types of infections. Energetic testing methods and applied kinesiology have typically been thought of as quackery by the conventional medical community; however, clinical evidence has proven this type of testing to be very effective.

In applied kinesiology, the practitioner detects infections by testing the patient's muscle response to different microbes. The strength of the muscle response helps the practitioner to determine whether that organism is present in the body. Different muscles of the body can be used for the test, although the arm muscles are most commonly used. Generally, testing involves the patient raising his or her arm, as the practitioner applies pressure to it. A homeopathic preparation of the microbe, or its energetic signature, or the suspected offending toxin, is concurrently placed somewhere within the vicinity of the patient. The patient is then asked to resist as the practitioner applies pressure to his/her arm. The degree to which the patient is able to resist indicates to the practitioner whether the particular microbe that has been placed on or near the patient is also present in the body, and to what degree. Practitioners can also test for the usefulness of different remedies by placing them within the vicinity of the patient and testing the patient's muscle response to them.

It's important to note that the usefulness of muscle testing depends upon several factors, including the competency of the tester, whether test samples exist for all the types of parasitic organisms that need to be tested for, and whether symptoms of infection are present in the tester (if the tester is ill, the results of applied kinesiology, or muscle testing, may be inaccurate).

I have noticed that at times, though an infection is present in my body, if the infection isn't causing me symptoms at the time when I am being tested, I will test negative for that infection via an applied kinesiology technique. Yet this doesn't mean that the microbes that have caused that infection aren't present and able to cause symptoms later on. It can be difficult to discern through applied kinesiology whether the infections will continue to be a problem for the body and cause symptoms once they have been brought under control. However, it isn't realistic to eliminate every pathogenic organism from the body. Living with some level of infection may be acceptable, as long as the infection isn't causing symptoms and the immune system is able to keep it under control so that it doesn't further damage the body.

Fortunately, other unconventional yet effective strategies exist for testing parasites. Among these are the Acupuncture Meridian Assessment test, also known as electrodermal screening (EDS); electro-acupuncture according to Dr. Reinhold Voll (EAV), and electro-acupuncture biofeedback. These tests measure energy flow through the body's meridians (its energy pathways). Changes in electrical conductivity at any one of the body's meridian points above or outside of what is considered to be normal indicates the possible presence of an infection in those parts of the body to which the particular meridian is connected.

Other bioenergetic testing devices, such as the ZYTO™, can also potentially detect parasites and other microbes by measuring energetic changes within the body and detecting energetic frequencies that correlate with the energetic frequencies of different microbes. Every living organism has a specific and measurable energetic frequency. Devices such as the ZYTO™ can detect the body's response to these frequencies. Bioenergetic testing should be combined with other methods of diagnosis. As with all types of testing methods, its use hasn't been perfected.

Another way to confirm whether parasites are causing symptoms is by doing an empirical trial of a broad-spectrum treatment that is designed to eliminate multiple types of parasites. Most chronically ill people have some parasites, as evidenced by the Herxheimer (detoxification) reactions that occur when they do parasite cleanses. Many of the problems in Lyme disease and chronic health conditions are vague and difficult to test for. Empirical trials are often needed to determine a patient's response to any given treatment methodology.

The only drawback to empirical trials is that they may not be able to provide information about which specific infections are present in the body. Applied kinesiology techniques and bioenergetic testing methods may be more useful for this purpose. Practitioners can determine not only which microbes are present, but the exact treatments, and how many, or much of them, a patient needs at a given time. Not everyone with the same set of parasitic infections will respond to the same treatments. Bioenergetic testing can reveal to the practitioner which treatments a patient needs, based on his or her biochemistry.

Anti-Parasitic Treatment

Many natural as well as pharmaceutical remedies can be used to treat parasites. The appropriate combination of remedies depends upon the person's biochemistry and ability to tolerate treatments, as well as the overall pathogen load and types of parasites present. Treatment must be individualized; a generalized protocol cannot be recommended for everyone. Dr. Yu, at the 2011 conference "A Deep Look Beyond Lyme," as well as in his 2010 book *Accidental Cure: Extraordinary Medicine for Extraordinary Patients*, noted that all of the herbal remedies and pharmaceutical medications listed below are useful for eliminating many types of parasites.

Herbal Remedies

- Black walnut hull extract
- Wormwood
- Clove oil
- Artemisia annua
- Citrus seed extract
- Pumpkin seed
- Ginger root
- Gentian root
- Goldenseal root
- Mimosa pudica (an Ayurvedic herb thought to be extremely potent, and more effective than many drugs for removing some types of parasites)

Pharmaceutical Medications

- Mebendazole
- Albendazole
- Metronidazole
- Praziquantel
- Iodoquinol
- Tinidazole
- Ivermectin
- Tetracycline/doxycycline
- Pyrental pamoate
- Nitazoxanide (Alinia)

Ann Louise Gittleman's book *Guess What Came To Dinner?* contains a comprehensive chart that lists the many different types of parasites found in humans, along with pharmaceutical remedies for each. Her book also contains a list of herbal cures that can be used for some types of infections. While this book was last updated in 2001, the information is comprehensive and still among the most relevant today.

Supportive Treatments

In addition to removing parasites from the body with herbs and medications, it's important to correct the underlying problems that allowed the parasites to gain a foothold in the body in the first place, to prevent new parasites from causing symptoms by returning to the body via common exposure routes. Healing involves replenishing nutrients, removing other environmental toxins such as heavy metals and pesticides, and correcting the systemic dysfunction caused by toxins and other infections.

Preventing the Return of Parasites

As previously mentioned, parasites are transmitted principally via food and water, as well as through animals, soil, and fecal matter. Once they have been removed from the body, it's important to avoid their return by doing all of the following:

1. Cooking and washing food thoroughly. Tapeworm comes from uncooked beef and pork. It can be easily avoided by thoroughly cooking meat.

2. Using a carbon block or reverse osmosis water filtering system that removes cysts and other microorganisms from tap water. *Giardia lamblia* is the most common water-borne parasitic infection (although it can be transmitted many different ways) in the United States. Once inside the body, it can significantly damage the GI tract, especially the villi that line the small intestine. Vitamin and mineral deficiencies then occur, as a result of the body not being able to properly absorb and assimilate nutrients. While the initial symptoms of *Giardia* are typically gastrointestinal, over time, chronic fatigue and depression can result from long-standing infections.

3. Washing hands thoroughly after using the bathroom or changing a baby's diaper, as parasites can be transmitted via fecal matter. Avoid

sitting on toilet seats in public places (and on your own if you don't clean them regularly).

4. Using gloves when working in the garden, and not walking barefoot outdoors on dirt or soil, since soil contains parasitic organisms.

5. Doing a parasite cleanse once or twice a year, after extensive treatment for the initial infections has been completed. Parasite cleanses usually involve taking multiple anti-parasitic herbs, such as wormwood, black walnut, clove, and Artemisia, in a combination tincture, capsule, or other form. Parasite cleanse products are sometimes sold as a package and include (in addition to herbs that remove parasites) pre- and probiotic products to replenish healthy bacteria in the gut, along with gut-healing substances such as L-glutamine, butyrate, slippery elm, and marshmallow root. (The latter are described in greater detail in the following chapter). Some popular cleansing products include: ReNew Life's ParaGone (www.renewlife.com/paragone.html), Parastroy™ from Nature's Secret (naturessecret.com/products/parastroy), and Humaworm (http://humaworm.com).

6. Taking a hydrochloric acid supplement if stomach acid levels are low, since stomach acid acts as a strong first line of defense against parasitic organisms.

In Summary

Parasite removal, as with Lyme disease treatment, can be a difficult and lengthy process. Parasites are adaptable and tenacious, as are Lyme organisms, and can sometimes evade pharmaceutical and herbal regimens. Yet removing them is important for a full recovery from chronic illness. They not only steal the body's nutrients, but also cause illness, which can be just as, if not more, severe than the illness caused by tick-borne infections. Removing them also makes it easier for the body to fight tick-borne infections, and to heal from other conditions of chronic illness.

Chapter Seven

Gastrointestinal Dysfunction

Gastrointestinal (GI) problems, such as dysbiosis (an imbalance in the amount of healthy bacteria in the gut compared to pathogenic bacteria), irritable bowel, and leaky gut syndrome are another main cause of serious chronic illness in people with Lyme disease. GI dysfunction may result from biochemical abnormalities induced by tick-borne infections, or it may be the reason that Lyme infections gain a foothold in the body in the first place. GI dysfunction leads to metabolic and immune system weakness that leaves the body susceptible to infections and disease. According to Jon Barron, a well-known alternative health expert and researcher, whose website attracts millions of visitors monthly and who is also the founder of the Baseline of Health® Foundation (www.jonbarron.org) and author of the book *Lessons from the Miracle Doctors*, "Many researchers now believe that declining levels of friendly bacteria in the intestinal tract may actually mark the onset of chronic, degenerative disease."

While gastrointestinal problems in some people with Lyme disease may be directly caused by tick-borne infections, other factors, such as declining levels of healthy bacteria in the gut also cause GI dysfunction. Conventionally raised meat and produce contain pesticides, hormones, antibiotics, and other toxins, all of which destroy the gut in various ways, as do environmental toxins and processed food, the latter of which contains lots of harmful additives and preservatives. Antibiotics wipe out beneficial bacteria in the gut that are meant to defend against incoming pathogens that enter the body through food and water. Pesticides, non-steroidal anti-inflammatory drugs, and chlorine in water, among other man-made toxins, also kill off beneficial gut bacteria and damage the villi (the little fingerlike projections in the small intestine involved in nutrient assimilation).

Joseph Mercola, MD, in an October, 12, 2011 article on his website, www. mercola.com, writes: "Virtually anything that can upset the balance of bacteria in your digestive tract can encourage damage to your intestinal lining that can lead to leaky gut. It's a very fragile system, and it's important to realize that your gut bacteria are very vulnerable to lifestyle and environmental factors." He then provides a chart of substances that damage the gut, which include (but are not limited to): processed foods, antibiotics, pollution, agricultural chemicals and pesticides; sugar, refined grains, and chlorinated and fluoridated water.

Doctors Rajendra Sharma (MB, B.Ch, BAO, MF Hom, MRCH) and Gloria Gilber (ND, DA Hom, PhD) on their website, *Leaky Gut Syndrome,* (www.leakygut.co.uk) cite antibiotics, pesticides, herbicides, fungicides and insecticides as among the most important contributing factors to leaky gut syndrome, a condition whereby the intestinal lining becomes inflamed and the villi, which produce enzymes and secretions essential for healthy nutrient absorption, become damaged or altered.

Viruses, bacteria, fungi, and parasites also harm the gut. They enter the body through the food we eat, the water we drink, and the air we breathe. The healthy bacteria that live in the gastrointestinal tract are the body's first line of defense against the millions of harmful organisms that enter it daily. According to Jon Barron, if the gut is in good condition, its healthy gut bacteria will neutralize most of the pathogens (up to 70 percent) that enter the body through food, water, and air. That said, these pathogenic organisms are able to gain a foothold in the body and cause symptoms if the gut isn't in good condition, and the more than 400 species of beneficial bacteria that we are born with have been destroyed by antibiotics, a poor diet, and environmental toxins. Antibiotics are especially harmful. Their prolonged use can wipe out most species of bacteria in the gut, many of which cannot be replaced with supplemental probiotics. According to Barron, 99 percent of the gut flora is comprised of just a small handful of bacterial species, most of which can be found in supplemental probiotic products. Yet little research exists on how important the remaining 300-some species are, and whether prolonged antibiotic use can permanently eliminate them. If these species are missing, the consequences for the body are unknown, but are important to discover, since the gut bacteria comprise the body's first line of defense against disease and are an important component of the immune system. The fact that many researchers now believe that GI problems set the stage for a whole range of degenerative autoimmune diseases should cause us to seriously question whether we should allow antibiotics into our bodies in the first place.

While it may be necessary for some people with Lyme disease to take antibiotics, those who decide to take them should be aware that by doing so, they are delivering a significant blow to their immune system. Of course, if tick-borne infections are ravaging the body or creating a life-threatening situation for the infected person, it may be better for that person to take antibiotics. Natural antimicrobial remedies such as herbs may be insufficient for bringing the infections under control. The decision to weaken one of the body's main defenses against pathogenic organisms—temporarily or perhaps even permanently—must be carefully weighed against the decision to remove dangerous infectious organisms that, without antibiotic therapy, could also cause severe, permanent damage to the body.

Personally, I believe that people who have severe symptoms caused primarily by tick-borne organisms may require aggressive and prolonged antibiotic therapy. At the same time, I have seen some people become more ill—irreversibly—after doing prolonged antibiotic therapy. Perhaps the antibiotics further weakened their immune system by destroying the healthy flora in their bodies. Alternatively, they may have been prescribed improper treatment regimens, had severe detoxification problems, or a weakened immune system that wasn't strong enough to mount an effective response against the pathogenic organisms.

My Experience with Antibiotic Therapy

While I believe that it was necessary for me to take antibiotics to effectively treat the tick-borne infections in my body, the drugs caused some negative side effects that persisted for a couple of years following my therapy. A few of those side effects remain with me to this day. They include blurriness in my right eye, a severely disrupted circadian rhythm, insomnia, and weight gain. The year that I took antibiotics, I also noticed signs of accelerated aging, which natural treatments didn't seem to produce. Still, I currently believe that the benefits of eliminating the infections outweighed the costs of using multiple drugs for over a year.

The decision about whether to take pharmaceutical antibiotics for tick-borne infections can be a challenging one. I took a completely natural approach to treating Lyme disease during the first five years that I was sick, and found it to be insufficient. But this may have been because my treatment regimen was inadequate, and I didn't have much personal guidance from Lyme-literate doctors about how to effectively use natural remedies. When I finally decided to take oral antibiotics, in conjunction with multiple herbal remedies, my pathogen load significantly decreased, although I didn't feel much better by the end of the treatment. This is probably because I hadn't yet adequately addressed the other causes of illness in my body. I still believe that antibiotic therapy was important, because I knew that the pathogens were destroying my body.

It may be wise for people who suspect that their symptoms aren't primarily caused by *Borrelia* and other tick-borne infections, or whose symptoms aren't severe, to consider a natural approach to treating tick-borne infections first. Perhaps they would benefit from using herbal remedies in conjunction with electromagnetic or biophoton treatments. Lee Cowden, MD, has an excellent herbal treatment protocol for Lyme disease that works well for some people. This protocol is described in greater detail on an Ecuadorian website under the heading "Cowden Support Program" (www.nutramedix.ec).

How Toxic Food Destroys the Gastrointestinal Tract

Toxic food also causes gastrointestinal problems by damaging gut villi. When the villi are damaged, the body's ability to absorb nutrients from food becomes compromised. Nutrients are fuel for the body and its rebuilding and regeneration processes. Vitamins, minerals, carbohydrates, fats, and protein, are the substances upon which new proteins are built, energy is created, and metabolic processes are carried out. If the body lacks any of these nutrients due to faulty micronutrient absorption, and instead receives toxins, every single organ, system, and tissue will cease to function properly.

In a person who has a healthy gut, most digestion takes place in the mouth and stomach. If the body is healthy and receives food in its natural state, digestion tends to be efficient. All raw, natural and unprocessed food contains all of the enzymes that are needed by the GI tract to digest it. Cooked, processed and refined food, as well as food that has been genetically modified, or had antibiotics, hormones, pesticides, and other harmful substances added to it no longer contains the enzymes that are required for digestion. The body has to work harder to digest such food by secreting greater amounts of hydrochloric acid and pancreatic enzymes, both of which are involved in digestion. This puts a tremendous stress upon the body, especially the pancreas, which may already be stressed because it has to contend with blood sugar imbalances caused by chronic illness.

Most people with Lyme disease have some degree of insulin resistance, a condition in which the cells become resistant to insulin, a hormone that brings glucose into the cells. This causes the pancreas, which produces insulin, to have to work harder to get this fuel to the body. Thus, the body uses up a lot of its energy to digest non-natural foods—energy that would be better used to recover from chronic illness. Despite the attempts of the GI tract to break down this bad food, much of it nonetheless ends up undigested in the small intestine. Normally, by the time food reaches the small intestine, it has been broken down enough for the small intestine to be able to effectively finish the digestion process and transfer the resultant nutrients to the bloodstream through the villi. If the body has been given enzymatically deficient, toxic food, large particles of undigested food and toxins end up in the villi. The villi are damaged by these toxins, which then end up in the bloodstream and cause inflammation and allergic reactions throughout the body.

Healing the Gut

Consuming food in an as natural a form as possible is important for healing the gut. Some nutritionists advocate a raw foods diet, contending that beneficial enzymes in the food get destroyed when food is cooked, which then makes the food harder to digest. This may be true; however, I have personally found cooked food (especially vegetables) to be easier to assimilate than raw food. The body appears to need more energy to digest raw food; energy that a chronically ill person may not be able to spare.

It may also be helpful to take digestive enzymes with meals, since enzymes aid the body in breaking down proteins, fats, and carbohydrates. Products that contain amylase, protease, lipase, and bromelain are best, since each of these plays a unique role in digestion. Amylase breaks down starches into sugar; protease and bromelain break down proteins into polypeptides and amino acids, and lipases break down fats. Taking supplemental ox bile may be beneficial if you have difficulty digesting fats, or have had your gall-bladder removed. Supplemental digestive enzymes also cause the pancreas and stomach to secrete lesser amounts of digestive juices. This reduces the energy that they must expend in the digestive process. Enzymes also help the body to more effectively break down food for assimilation by the small intestine, and leave the body with more energy for other purposes, such as immune function.

Chewing food thoroughly also helps the GI tract to break down and assimilate nutrients, since saliva contains digestive enzymes. Enzymatic digestion begins in the mouth, not the stomach. The more you chew your food, the easier it will be for the gut to further digest that food.

If gut health has been compromised by years of toxins, stress, poor dietary habits, and infections, it's also important to heal the intestinal lining with remedies such as slippery elm, L-glutamine, aloe vera, and marshmallow root. All of these substances work to heal the gut in various ways: by reducing inflammation, soothing mucous membrane tissue, improving immune function, and eliminating pathogens.

Aloe vera contains polysaccharides, which have an anti-inflammatory effect upon gut lining, and antimicrobial properties that may help to eliminate pathogens from the GI tract. It is also an important immune system modulator.

Slippery elm soothes the gut through its anti-oxidative effects upon gut tissue, and provides mucilage, which coats and protects the intestinal lining from toxins and pathogenic organisms.

Marshmallow root is another herb that contains mucilage. It also reduces inflammation and aids the body in expelling excess mucus, and improves immune system function by stimulating phagocytosis, a process in which cells called macrophages engulf and digest infectious microorganisms that cause disease.

Finally, L-glutamine is the primary fuel for all of the digestive cells. It is very effective at healing an inflamed or damaged digestive tract.

Butyric acid is a beneficial substance for healing the colon, since it repairs and regenerates colonic epithelial cells (those which line the colon). Butyric acid is produced by bacteria in the colon through the fermentation of fiber and starch. Taking fiber supplements and eating a high-fiber diet is a good way to increase butyric acid production. Colon cleanses also promote healing of the large intestine by removing toxins that have accumulated there over time.

Taking a quality probiotic product is important for re-inoculating the gut with beneficial bacteria that have been destroyed by toxins and antibiotics. It helps to restore immune function and the body's defenses against pathogenic bacteria.

The gut contains hundreds of species of bacteria, although some experts believe that only thirty to forty comprise the majority, so it may be ideal to look for a probiotic product that contains as many species as possible. Researched Nutritionals® (www.researchednutritionals.com), makes a product called Prescript-Assist Pro™, which contains over thirty types of soil-based bacterial organisms. According to the Researched Nutritionals website, "SBOs are soil-based probiotic organisms found in healthy soils, which produce and release powerful enzymes that prepare and purify soil to support plant growth. Natural soil is a living biomass composed of SBO's, fungi, yeasts, and microscopic insects. The role of SBO's is to keep the soil biomass in a healthy, dynamic balance that supports the growth of plants and animals. Additionally, SBO's simultaneously produce and release specific nutrients necessary to accelerate plant development and reproduction. SBO's play the same role in the gut as they do in the soil: supporting the healthy growth of organisms."

Soil-based organisms secrete enzymes that rid the intestinal tract of pathogenic organisms. They also have other beneficial effects upon the body, such as metabolizing proteins for the cells, helping the cells to rid the body of toxic waste, and increasing the overall absorption of nutrients.

In addition to Researched Nutritionals' Prescript-Assist Pro, a few other reputable companies produce quality probiotic products, whose effectiveness has been backed by scientific research: Klaire Labs® (www.klaire.com), VSL#3 (www.vsl3.com), and Custom Probiotics Inc. (www.customprobiotics.com).

While it may be beneficial to look for probiotic products that contain a wide variety of bacteria, according to Jon Barron, only a few types of these bacteria have been extensively researched and their benefits validated. Among these are L. acidophilus and bifidobacteria. L. acidophilus produces many compounds that inhibit the growth of nearly two dozen disease-causing pathogenic organisms. Bifidobacteria also produce B-vitamins and eliminate many cancer-causing elements from the body. Other strains of bacteria may also improve immune function, but of all the types of bacteria that have been studied, L. acidophilus and bifidobacteria are currently thought to be most important for gut health.

As previously mentioned, it's important to choose a probiotic product that contains live organisms. Studies have revealed that many of the so-called live bacteria in probiotic products are dead within several months after the products' manufacture. Heat and moisture accelerate this process. For this reason, it's important to choose a probiotic product that has received high ratings based on user experience, not simply laboratory testing at the time of manufacture.

It's also essential to incorporate probiotic-containing foods into the diet. Such foods may include: yogurt, kefir (a fermented dairy product, similar in texture and flavor to yogurt); kimchi (a traditional fermented Korean dish made from vegetables and a variety of seasonings); sauerkraut, kombucha (a fermented Asian tea); miso soup (a Japanese soup made from fermented rye, soybeans, rice, or barley); microalgae (such as spirulina, chlorella, and blue-green algae), and even dark chocolate (without sugar!). Consuming some, or all, of these foods on a regular basis can help to replenish the beneficial bacteria that protect the body against disease-causing pathogens.

Cow and goat's milk yogurt are naturally rich sources of probiotics, but U.S. law requires that all commercial dairy products be pasteurized. Pasteurization destroys vital digestive enzymes and beneficial bacteria in dairy products, thereby rendering them inflammatory to the body and useless as probiotic sources (unless the bacteria are added back into the yogurt after pasteurization, which they often are). Fortunately, raw cow and goat's dairy products can still be purchased directly from some farms. This may be a better choice for people with health challenges. Alternatively, most people can consume kimchi, sauerkraut, and some of the other aforementioned probiotic foods without suffering adverse effects to their health. Coconut kefir may also be a healthy alternative to dairy kefir products, although many coconut yogurt and kefir products also contain cane sugar and carrageenan (a harmful food additive), so it's important to find ones that don't.

In Summary

Gastrointestinal dysfunction is a major contributing factor to chronic illness in people with tick-borne infections. It may even be a primary cause of disease. For this reason, gut health should not be treated as an incidental or subsidiary component of recovery. Healing the GI tract is just as essential as ridding the body of tick-borne infections. The health of the gut ultimately impacts every system and organ of the body. Whenever GI tract function is compromised by pathogenic organisms, toxins, antibiotics, damaged villi and other factors, it cannot effectively break down, assimilate, and utilize nutrients from food. This results in nutrient deficiencies, infections, and inflammation throughout the body.

Much of the immune system resides in the gut, so it's important to heal it and make sure that it's functioning as effectively as possible. This involves: 1) removing the fungal, viral, parasitic, and bacterial infections there;

2) maintaining a natural, organic, non-allergenic diet; 3) facilitating the digestive process by chewing food well, taking enzymes and hydrochloric acid (if stomach levels are low); 4) removing toxins from the diet and one's environment, and avoiding future exposure to antibiotics, GMOs, and harmful industrial contaminants which are used on food crops, such as pesticides, herbicides, and fungicides; and 5) healing the gut with natural substances such as marshmallow root and butyrate, probiotics and soil-based microorganisms. Finally, patients and practitioners who treat tick-borne infections with antibiotics should realize that it may be counterproductive to do round after round of antibiotic therapy if no measures are also simultaneously undertaken to heal the gut. Doctors who give their patients multiple oral antibiotics without also prescribing probiotics and other gut-healing substances fail to understand the negative impact that antibiotics have upon the body, and the important role of the gut in healing the body.

Chapter Eight

Emotional Trauma and Depression

Many people tend to view Lyme disease and chronic illness as the result of infections and environmental toxins. They contend that these are what break the immune system. But what if a broken immune system allowed the infections and toxins to cause symptoms in the first place? What if the root of the problem is the immune system, and the infections and toxicity are simply the branches that stem from this bad root?

Even people with strong immune systems can tolerate the onslaught of only so much environmental garbage, but when the immune system is weak to begin with, it will tolerate very little, or nothing at all. It will react to every sneeze, bug, perfume, and genetically modified food on the planet, and I'm not sure that avoiding every irritant is the way to health. A weak immune system will spend its life in overdrive, responding to every animal hair and pathogen that crosses its path. And the person with the weak immune system will never truly get well, except temporarily and/or unless shrouded in a perfectly uncontaminated environment, the likes of which don't exist on our planet.

We are poisoning ourselves to death with all of the pollution we have created, with the superbugs, uranium contamination, GMOs, and so on. Yet eliminating contaminants from the body and removing infectious agents may only bring the immune system back to the sputtering, yet moderately functional "square one" state that it was in before being assaulted with all of the environmental garbage.

To heal the immune system, it's important to know what caused it to malfunction before it was weakened by tick-borne infections. It's also vital to understand whether tick-borne infections and toxins were the primary cause of its downfall, or whether another factor rendered it unable to fight the toxins and pathogens in the first place. Yes, sometimes pathogens and environmental pollutants are primarily the cause of its malfunctioning. I believe that people who were strong and healthy prior to getting Lyme disease have had their immune systems hamstrung mostly by infections, particularly when the strains of *Borrelia* and the mix of co-infections that they contracted were especially virulent. But there is another camp of people—those who have had a lifelong history of cold viruses, allergies, asthma, pain, fatigue, depression and other health problems—whose immune systems were never that strong to begin with. Such people are predisposed to sickness from tick-borne infections, but the tick-borne infections aren't the main reason for their illnesses.

Knowing the primary cause of immune dysfunction matters, even though the toxins and infections must be removed anyway. If it wasn't these things that caused immune dysfunction in the first place, it's important to find out what did, so that the underlying cause of that dysfunction can be treated.

Some doctors use immune modulators to try to restore their patients' immune systems. Medicinal mushrooms and colostrum, which boost natural killer (NK) cell counts, are popular remedies for people with Lyme, since NK cell counts tend to be low in this population. Beta 1,3 glucans, which help to regulate immune function, are also frequently used to treat chronic illness and may produce positive results in those who take them.

Yet immune function isn't just affected by what we ingest or by our physical environment. Sometimes the immune system refuses to heal, even when toxins are removed and infections are brought mostly under control. When eliminating infections, removing toxins, and supporting the body prove to be insufficient for healing, it may be because the immune system was damaged early on in life by other stressors—especially, and most commonly, emotional trauma. When this is the case, strengthening and healing the immune system requires identifying and healing that trauma.

Many studies have shown that emotional trauma causes physical illness. A January 2011 article in *Frontiers in Developmental Psychology* states that:

> "The experience of traumatic events in childhood has consequences for health in adulthood. A broad range of traumatic events experienced in childhood including physical abuse, sexual abuse, prolonged hospitalization, and family instability such as parental unemployment or substance abuse have been linked to chronic illness in adulthood stemming from poor immune functioning or poor cardiovascular health."

Trauma produces pro-inflammatory cytokines that damage the body. If prolonged and chronic, the body breaks down as a result of this inflammation, and disease results.

Ray Sahelian, MD, bestselling author of the book *Mind Boosters*, writes in an online article, "Clinical and experimental studies indicate that stress and depression are associated with the up-regulation of the immune system, including increased production of pro-inflammatory cytokines."

In another article, "Why Trauma Makes People Sick: Inflammation, Heart Disease and Diabetes in Trauma Survivors," health psychologist Kathleen A. Kendall-Tackett, PhD, writes:

> "Trauma survivors have higher than average rates of serious illness including heart disease, diabetes and metabolic syndrome, the precursor to type 2 diabetes. The intriguing question is why this is so. One possible explanation is the connection between disease and inflammation—specifically, elevated levels of pro-inflammatory cytokines. Cytokines are proteins that regulate immune response and pro-inflammatory cytokines help the body heal wounds and fight infection. But there can be too much of a good thing; chronic inflammation is a likely cause of a wide range of illnesses including heart disease, diabetes, Alzheimer's disease, and even cancer."

Bernie Siegel, MD, in his NY Times bestselling book, *Love, Medicine and Miracles,* estimates that 80 percent of his (former) cancer patients were either unwanted or treated indifferently as children. He writes that happy people are generally healthy people, and that it is love that creates health in the body. People who have suffered from severe emotional trauma and felt unloved or unwanted by their primary caregivers often become vulnerable to disease later in life.

Our Beliefs and Thoughts Control Our Biology

Emotional trauma causes unhealthy immune responses and disease because it tends to create unhealthy beliefs, thoughts, and behaviors in the afflicted, which then also affects the health of the body. In his book *The Biology of Belief,* scientist and bestselling author Bruce Lipton, PhD, contends that our thoughts emanate specific energetic frequencies throughout our cells, which affect our DNA and, in turn the health of our bodies—for better or worse. In his book, he writes, "Thoughts, the mind's energy, directly influence how the physical brain controls the body's physiology. Thought 'energy' can activate or inhibit the cell's function-producing proteins via the mechanics of constructive and destructive interference." From his research, Dr. Lipton has learned that nearly every major illness that people acquire has been linked to chronic stress. Furthermore, Lipton contends that ". . . harnessing the power of your mind (to change your thoughts, and consequently, your biology) can be more effective than the drugs you have been programmed to believe you need."

Other researchers have come to similar conclusions about the mind's power to alter the biochemistry. For example, the Japanese author Masaru Emoto, in his book, *The Hidden Messages in Water*, described a series of experiments in which specific thoughts were directed at water just before it was frozen. He observed that certain crystal patterns would emerge in the frozen water, according to the type of thought that was projected. For instance, water that had been exposed to loving words resulted in brilliant, colorful snowflake patterns, whereas water that had been exposed to negative thoughts formed incomplete, asymmetrical patterns with dull colors. And our bodies are about 70 percent water!

What we believe, think, and do on a daily basis has powerful ramifications for our health. For many people, disease starts in the soul and spirit then works its way outward to the body. I have met healthcare professionals who believe that disease is almost always a spiritual problem, but also others who claim that it plays only a minor role in the development of illness. Yet others (possibly a majority) believe that both physical toxins and infections, along with emotional/spiritual wounds, cause disease.

My perspective is that you can't live in a cesspool of environmental toxicity and survive, but neither can you expect to be healthy if anger, depression, sadness, and/or anxiety, all of which result from trauma, are your habitual state of being. In speaking with hundreds of chronically ill people, and examining my own experience with disease, I believe that emotional trauma is a primary cause of illness in many people with Lyme disease. Environmental toxins and pathogens simply cause symptoms in a body that is already predisposed to disease.

I have also observed that physicians (even holistic doctors), and their chronically ill patients, treat emotional trauma as just another ancillary problem that needs to be dealt with along with hormones, diet, and the like. Many people know that their thinking and beliefs aren't healthy, or that the way they live isn't healthy, but they pay greater attention to their diets or to their antibiotic remedies than to the destructive habits and thinking patterns that are the root of their diseases.

It can be difficult to focus on healing the soul or emotional trauma when doctors, family members, and most of society contends that what you really need to pay attention to are the bugs, the biofilm, and the bad water you're drinking. All of these things matter, but healing trauma should not be relegated to an adjunct component of recovery. It is, for many, absolutely primary.

The Challenge of Healing Unhealthy Beliefs, Thoughts, and Behaviors

One of the most important aspects of healing trauma involves changing the unhealthy beliefs, thoughts, and behavioral patterns that have resulted from that trauma. Unlike taking a drug or vitamin, however, this isn't a thirty-second, three-times-per-day activity. It requires a minute-by-minute, day-by-day awareness of your thoughts and activities. It is a full-time job. Most of us don't pursue healing our inner wounds as intensely as we could, because it can be a tremendous, difficult responsibility. Few people—never mind incredibly sick people—are up for the challenge. We would rather take fifty pills a day for years, and suffer a decade of Herxheimer reactions than attempt to change the way we think and live. For some, taking two hundred supplements, spending thousands of dollars per year on treatments, and living for years in physical and emotional pain, is easier than changing a lifetime of bad mental programming. Truly, I think that subconsciously this is what some of us believe.

Or we may think, *what's the use, anyway?* We spend a half an hour per day on meditation, visit counselors, and practice strategies for gratitude, and yet, the soul sickness persists. We reason that once we get rid of the infections and toxins in our bodies, we will be happy. Our thoughts and behaviors will change for the better, because our brains and bodies will be healthier.

And this may be true. Pathogens and toxins cause depression, fatigue, anxiety, irritability, brain fog, and pain. This, along with the financial hardship and life of isolation that tend to beset the chronically ill, make it incredibly difficult to focus upon changing unhealthy thoughts or habits, or the original cause of trauma that opened the door to symptoms. The odds are stacked to skyscraper dimensions against the chronically ill person. However, the sad paradox of disease is that sometimes the body will not heal until the trauma is dealt with. It's a difficult catch-22. The sick need nutrition and cleansing, along with financial and emotional support, in order to have the willpower, stamina, and clarity of mind to pursue healing of the soul. Yet the wounded soul must also be healed if the body is to heal. Treatments will not be sufficient.

Revelation, or Awareness, Is Half the Battle

On the bright side, sickness can positively motivate some people to pursue inner healing, when they realize that the health of their souls is integral to the health of their bodies. Desperation prompts some people to somehow find it within themselves to revamp their entire lives, even when the odds are stacked against them.

Adopting healthier patterns of thought and behavior isn't accomplished overnight, but it happens faster when you finally realize that your depression isn't just caused by your symptoms, or by a life of isolation, but also by the way you have lived and what you have believed for years prior to becoming ill. Healing moves at an accelerated rate when you truly understand that it's not "all about the bugs," and you commit to the healing of your soul as powerfully as you commit to the eradicating of infections and physical toxins.

Revelation knowledge can be a mighty motivator when sickness conspires against the ability to do little more than swallow a few pills to get well. You may find the strength within to change the toxic thoughts and behaviors that made you sick in the first place when you understand that the prescription you need is forgiveness; of yourself, others, and God. When you realize that sunshine and laughter will do more for your immune system than a vitamin. When finding peace becomes more important than finding the next remedy. In short, when you stop believing the lie that happiness resides only in healing the body and not the soul.

I have learned these truths through my own experience of healing from emotional trauma. My personal relationship with God, in particular, has been instrumental in teaching me how to establish healthier beliefs and behaviors. I haven't perfectly implemented what I have learned. I still have workaholic tendencies, borne out of a lack of trust that I will be provided for, especially during times of illness when I have been unable to work, and a mental stronghold of performance orientation. I also struggle to overcome negative thinking, because it has been my mind's pattern since early childhood. The habit isn't broken easily. Thankfully, I am mostly aware when my thoughts aren't healthy, and I am able to continually remind myself of better ways of being and thinking. But that said, I am still learning to implement what I know.

The Link between Emotional Trauma and Depression

Depression results from unhealthy beliefs, thoughts, and behaviors, and can be challenging to heal. In people with Lyme disease, this is a problem, since Lyme sufferers and their doctors may mistakenly assume that the depression is due mostly to tick-borne infections and toxins. They believe that the depression will disappear with the infections or with the prescription of an antidepressant medication. If the root cause of depression, which is trauma, hasn't been dealt with, however, the depression is unlikely to abate with a prescription drug or by eliminating infections. It may not even be possible for some people to heal from Lyme if an underlying emotional stressor is perpetuating their depression, and consequently, disease-promoting inflammation.

Many practitioners and people with Lyme usually focus on treating symptoms of depression, along with the tick-borne infections, instead of addressing the underlying emotional trauma. Rather than dig up the roots of disease, they treat the branches. I believe that Lyme disease infections are, for some people, nothing more than branches; a manifestation of a deeper problem in the soul that requires healing. Carpet-bombing pathogens or doing a toxin-removal protocol puts out fires in the body (which is crucial once these fires have started!), but never gets to the arsonists that are starting the fires in the first place.

Thus, while it is important to remove infections and toxins, people whose depression is caused by other factors may also need to pursue strategies such as counseling, prayer, and meditation, in order to remove the unhealthy beliefs, thoughts, and behaviors that are perpetuating their condition. This, along with nutritional therapies that restore the brain's chemistry and support the development of new thoughts and behaviors, are essential for healing. Such strategies will be discussed in greater detail in the following sections.

Behavioral/Cognitive Strategies for Healing Emotional Trauma

I have studied the work of many healers, and discovered that healing trauma usually involves part or all of the following:

1. Forgiving people who have wronged us in the past. This does not mean agreeing with what they did, or "letting them off the hook." It is about freeing a prisoner—us—because we are the only ones harmed by our anger or rage toward others. The people we are mad at are usually unaware of how we feel, but choosing to forgive

them frees our minds and bodies from the toxic consequences of anger and resentment. Sometimes, we may not feel it in our hearts to forgive another person, but feelings can sometimes follow the decision to forgive. We usually assume that we have to change our feelings toward people before we can forgive them. But repeatedly acknowledging our desire to free them of the debt they owe us can, regardless of our feelings, enable our hearts to change toward them over time. Many healing ministers (myself included) have seen people miraculously freed from disease when, along with prayer, they chose to forgive someone who had profoundly wounded them.

2. Accessing and addressing the harmful beliefs and thought patterns that have resulted from abuse or trauma, and replacing those with healthy ones. This is not easy to do, and may require many months or years of diligent work with a trusted counselor, minister, or practitioner who is trained to discern and recognize the roots of harmful beliefs and thought patterns. The healer must also know how to effectively help the depressed person replace the lies that he or she has learned to believe, with positive truths. My experience has been that the voice of truth is always positive, empowering, and encouraging. It is never critical, judgmental, or discouraging. Once we grasp the reality of our immense value and importance in the world, we can learn to replace the negative tapes that play in our heads with positive ones, and healing can occur.

3. Discerning any subconscious motivations for disease, and replacing those with motivations for wellness. The subconscious desire to be ill often results from emotional trauma and believing lies about one-self (such as, *disease keeps me safe from the world and being rejected by it; I am not worthy of health; or, I can better help others if I am sick*).

Sarah Myhill is a British physician who specializes in chronic fatigue syndrome (or myalgic encephalomyelitis, as it is often referred to in the United Kingdom). She has treated over 4,500 patients with CFS. In an e-book, she writes about such blocks to healing: "Some people clearly want to get better, but there is some deep-seated reason, some unresolved psychological 'pain' which is blocking [their] possible improvement. Very often these patients don't know themselves [that] they have a block about getting better, and it may take a great deal of thought and honesty with themselves to identify 'blocking factors.' For example, once patients become ill and unable to care for themselves, they lose a certain amount of responsibility for their own lives. The thought of having to take responsibility again and the worry of not being 'reliably well' may provide a subconscious block to improvement. Psychologically, they cannot afford to get better. These people can be thought of as having a 'psychological disability' which is just as disabling and difficult to deal with as any physical disability."

You don't need to be ashamed if you discover that you have a subconscious block to healing. Such blocks are a normal response of the body and psyche to trauma, and are the soul's way of trying to protect itself. Yet it's important that these blocks be discerned and removed so that the body and mind can heal.

Once any subconscious motivations for sickness are discovered through a counselor, introspection, or by some other method, it's important to pursue and embrace higher truths, to replace the lies that were unintentionally birthed in the psyche, and begin acting on those truths. Often, people will continue to operate out of the lies residing in their subconscious minds until someone challenges them to think differently, and/or they can heal the wounds that caused those lies to become established in the mind.

4. Finding support and love within a community of people who can help you to live out what you have learned to be true about yourself, and who can help you to see a different reality than the one that caused you to become traumatized in the first place. For example, joining an organization that maintains as its foremost goal to love others and accept them unconditionally, regardless of beliefs, lifestyle, or other issues, may be one place where you can meet such people. People who truly understand unconditional love will embrace others without having expectations of them.

5. Some twelve-step recovery groups can be incredibly supportive and help people to heal from emotional trauma by teaching them

healthier ways of thinking and being (for example, Co-Dependents Anonymous). Members are encouraged to surrender their burdens to a higher power and to rely upon one another for help. Twelve-step groups may be an especially good option for those who don't feel comfortable in churches or within structured religious organizations.

6. Because chronic illness is challenging on multiple levels, it's vital to have more than just one person to count on and confide in for emotional support. Churches, twelve-step recovery, and other types of support groups (e.g., those for people with Lyme disease and other chronic illnesses) can sometimes provide this companionship and support. Some organizations may also offer low-key recreational activities, which can help people who are sick and disabled to shed their lives of isolation.

7. If you don't live with or near friends who can support you in your healing journey, then move. If the nearest loved one is 50 miles away, and you haven't found companionship with any of your neighbors or within an organization, consider changing your living situation. If you remain isolated, it can be more difficult to heal, especially if you notice that the isolation leaves you feeling depressed and lonely. If you can't get out of the house often because you are really sick, consider a community living situation with others who have similar health challenges or who understand such challenges. In any case, it's important to spend time with people who are positive and uplifting.

8. Have friends who talk about other topics besides sickness and symptoms—yours or theirs. Misery loves company, and while it can be tempting to spend time with people who are suffering in the same way as you, disease talk reinforces those challenges. Symptoms and treatments already clamor for your undivided attention—why give them more? We all need people to vent our suffering to, but sometimes, the most healing thing you can do is to ignore your soul's desire to complain, yet again, about how bad you feel. While it's imperative to have friends who understand your pain, over time,

talking about symptoms can become an addiction that prevents healing. The adage that we become what we focus on is often true.

9. Make a list of activities that you can do that you enjoy, which are healing for the mind, body, and spirit, and which have nothing to do with disease (for instance, not researching treatments). Then commit to doing at least one of these activities daily. Such activities may include watching a funny movie, walking in the sunshine, reading a novel on the beach, or taking up a hobby like painting or Pilates.

It's also important to understand that healing from trauma isn't just about reading an inspirational book, finding a few good friends, or praying for a half-hour daily. It's about identifying and changing lifelong thought patterns, beliefs, and behaviors that have contributed to disease, which is far more difficult than taking a pill or even enduring a Herxheimer (detoxification) reaction. Healing is about understanding, on a heart level, not just in the mind, that the deepest and most profound changes will occur as you attend to these aspects of your well-being. It's not enough to just mentally assent to the fact that your anger, shame, and lack of forgiveness are making you sick. The truth must also reach your heart in a revelatory manner if true change is to occur. Healing also requires a powerful commitment to get well.

You may believe this, but haven't been motivated to change your thoughts or behavior, because deep down, your hope is still mostly in medical treatments, or you feel too sick to make the necessary changes. If so, I recommend asking a trusted counselor, friend, practitioner or mentor for help, or praying for revelation about what you need to do to heal. Because it is revelation knowledge that provides the conviction for people to change the way they think and live, not mere agreement with principles. Then trust that this revelation will come, in one form or another.

Healing from the Effects of Performance-Orientation

Emotional trauma can sometimes cause people to place unrealistic expectations upon themselves, because they believe that they have to strive in order to survive. This is borne out of fear that unless they are super-achievers, they won't make it in the world or be loved. This belief is especially strong among those who had caregivers who inadvertently taught them that receiving love was contingent upon their behavior. It doesn't help that our society tends to assign worth and value to those who accomplish, and to those who are beautiful, intelligent, and get things done. As a society, we tend to believe that our worth comes from what we do, instead of who we are.

I have traveled to over fifty nations and lived in three countries besides the United States, and have observed that people in the United States tend to have high expectations in relationships, compared to people who live in less-developed societies. I surmise that this is due to our performance-oriented culture, which demands that we be engaging, interesting, intelligent, and in a good mood, at all times. Such expectations make us sick, because they are rooted in perfectionistic ideals. Gerald Poesnecker, ND, notes in his book *Chronic Fatigue Unmasked*, that perfectionism is a trait found in those with adrenal weakness and chronic fatigue syndrome, and that it contributes to immune suppression and what he calls "the Adrenal Syndrome."

When emotional trauma is healed, performance orientation ceases and people learn to value themselves not for what they can accomplish, but for who they are. They cease to strive in their daily activities and stop operating in "fight or flight mode." This in turn, enables the body to heal.

Getting Out of Isolation

Living in isolation is another byproduct of emotional trauma. Deeply wounded people tend to mistrust others and sometimes want to hide from society. Paradoxically, isolation also results from chronic illness, since sick people don't feel well enough to get out and be with others who may not understand what they are going through. It may be difficult for them to find others who won't judge or expect things of them when they feel poorly. While few people with raging symptoms feel like laughing it up or being with others who might drain them further with their own problems, sadly, isolation perpetuates depression and suppresses immune function.

Human beings are designed to live in community; to rely upon and share life with one another. We need to be understood by others. We need to provide for others, and be provided for by them. We need to laugh. We need to be held. We need to get out of our heads and forget our problems, which is easier to do in the company of others.

Spending time with people who don't understand chronic illness or who don't have a healthy sense of personal boundaries or respect for the boundaries of others is extremely draining for the chronically ill. (For more information on the concept of boundaries, I invite you to read Henry Cloud and John Townsend's excellent book series on the topic). However, we are meant to be with people. Getting out of isolation, however possible, is important for healing from depression and emotional trauma, especially if isolation is one of the manifestations of that trauma.

Releasing Stored Emotional Trauma from the Tissues and Organs

Memories and trauma aren't held exclusively in the brain, but in all the tissues and organs of the body. Different energetic treatments and therapies can access and release those stored memories, and sometimes facilitate emotional and physical healing.

Lyme-literate doctor Lee Cowden, MD, uses voice-analysis software called EVOX for this purpose. In my book, *Insights Into Lyme Disease Treatment: 13 Lyme-Literate Health Care Practitioners Share Their Healing Strategies,* Dr. Cowden states that the voice contains energetic frequencies that correspond to harmful emotions that are held in the body due to trauma. After a person's voice is recorded through the EVOX system, a homeopathic dilution of that voice recording can be made and delivered back to the person through a hand cradle on a computerized ZYTO device. The frequencies in the homeopathic remedy have the effect of "shifting" the person energetically, so that the cells release the trauma they were holding.

The Healing Code system of Alexander Loyd, ND, is another therapy that energetically releases trauma. Dr. Loyd discovered that holding the hands in certain positions around the face and head while repeating affirmations cancels out disease-causing energetic frequencies which emanate from the cells and which are caused by stored traumatic memories. Once the body no longer has to contend with these disease-causing frequencies, emotional and physical healing can ensue. This inexpensive method has apparently been very successful for some people, as evidenced by the multitude of positive reviews that the *The Healing Code* book has received on Amazon.com.

The Role of Nutrients and Hormones in Supporting Emotional Healing

While cognitive and behavioral strategies are important for healing trauma and depression, it's also crucial to maintain a healthy diet and take mood-supportive nutritional supplements to support the biochemistry. Bioidentical hormone replacement therapy may also be necessary for some. Supporting the body with nutrition and balancing the hormones and neurotransmitters can better equip people who have a history of trauma to attend to their unhealthy beliefs, thoughts, and behaviors, since the body's nutritional and hormonal status powerfully influence mood, thought and behavior.

Restoring Healthy Neurotransmitter Levels

Neurotransmitter deficiencies are often present in people with a history of emotional trauma and depression. Neurotransmitters are constructed in the body from amino acids, in conjunction with vitamin and mineral co-factors, and are heavily involved in regulating mood and mediating other symptoms of depression, such as fatigue and pain. NeuroScience, Inc. (www.neurorelief.com) has available fifteen different tests for measuring neurotransmitter levels and their activity in the body. Most depressed people are deficient in serotonin, and sometimes, dopamine, two of the brain's principal neurotransmitters involved in mood regulation.

Doctors of integrative and naturopathic medicine often prescribe amino acids such as 5-hydroxytryptophan (5-HTP) and L-tryptophan to increase serotonin in the body, and/or L-phenylalaline or L-tyrosine to increase dopamine. While sometimes effective, people with adrenal fatigue and/or methylation problems (which is many people with chronic illness and Lyme disease), don't always respond well to these amino acids, especially when they are given alone or in high-dose sophisticated formulations. The body requires nutrient cofactors to make neurotransmitters from amino acids and some people don't have sufficient levels of these cofactors or cannot effectively use them to synthesize neurotransmitters.

All of the following cofactors are required to make serotonin from 5-HTP:

- Magnesium
- Vitamin C
- Zinc
- Vitamin B-6

People with Lyme disease and chronic illness tend to be deficient in all of these nutrients. *Borrelia,* one of the principal microbes involved in Lyme disease, is thought to deplete magnesium and other nutrients from the body, so replacing these with pharmaceutical-grade supplements is important. Some studies have revealed that *Borrelia* utilizes magnesium to create biofilms, which are polysaccharide matrixes that envelope and protect microbes from antimicrobial treatments. Because of this, some doctors discourage magnesium supplementation, but the fact is, the body requires magnesium to function effectively. Other doctors believe that it's more important to give the body what it needs, so that the immune system can better fight disease, even if some of those nutrients are also used by the microorganisms.

As described in Chapter Five, 80 percent of people with Lyme disease, and 50 percent of those with depression, suffer from a condition called pyroluria, which causes severe zinc, vitamin B-6, and other nutrient deficiencies. Because both zinc and vitamin B-6 are needed to produce serotonin, it's no surprise that many people with Lyme disease—never mind those with a history of emotional trauma!—don't have enough happiness-inducing neurotransmitters. Correcting pyroluria by taking high doses of minerals and bioavailable B-6 can therefore help to heal depression and enable people with a history of trauma to think positive, healthy thoughts, by changing the body's chemistry.

It's important to note here that many people, especially the adrenally fatigued, cannot effectively utilize vitamin B-6 to make serotonin. Taking P-5-P (pyridoxal phosphate), a more bioavailable metabolite of vitamin B-6, along with L-cystine can help the body to more effectively convert 5-HTP into serotonin. (Note that there is another similarly named substance called L-cysteine, which is chemically similar to L-cystine, although a different amino acid than the one that I am referring to here).

The body can also make serotonin from the amino acid L-tryptophan, which is a precursor to 5-HTP. The cofactors required to do this are folate, iron, calcium, and vitamin B-3. Many people with tick-borne infections (especially women) are deficient in iron. Increasing iron levels is typically difficult until infections are effectively treated, since some infections, like *Babesia*, deplete iron from the body. Therefore, 5-HTP may be a better choice of amino acid for increasing serotonin than L-tryptophan. It is also one step closer to serotonin on the amino acid synthesis chain, so it may be easier for the body to make serotonin from L-tryptophan.

L-tryptophan is found in some foods, but levels of this amino acid are quickly depleted by the stress of chronic illness. Still, it may be beneficial to include some or all of the following L-trytophan-containing foods in the diet to increase serotonin, along with a supplemental L-tryptophan or 5-HTP product (no foods contain 5-HTP; the body must make this amino acid from tryptophan).

Foods that contain tryptophan:

- Turkey
- Cottage cheese
- Almonds
- Pumpkin seeds
- Tuna

By themselves, these foods are insufficient for healing depression, but can provide support on the road to recovery.

Increasing dopamine, another neurotransmitter responsible for regulating mood, may also be helpful for recovery. Mucuna bean powder, which is used as a primary treatment for Parkinson's in India, contains L-dopa, the immediate precursor to dopamine, and is a great supplement for increasing dopamine levels. It is also easier for the body to assimilate than L-phenylalaline and L-tyrosine, amino acids that are sometimes given to increase dopamine. It may also be a better choice than L-tyrosine for those prone to anxiety, since L-tyrosine can cause anxiety.

Brightly colored fruits and vegetables are high in antioxidants. Consuming these foods is another way to indirectly increase dopamine, as they help to neutralize free radicals that deplete dopamine in the body. Similarly, animal protein, beans, lentils, nuts, and seeds increase dopamine; however, as with foods containing L-tryptophan, they are, by themselves, probably insufficient to correct severe deficiencies.

Healing the Brain with Omega-3 Fatty Acids

Omega-3 fatty acids play a role in healing the body of depression. They support brain cell structure, increase neurotransmitter production, and reduce inflammation. They also heal brain and nervous tissue, which get destroyed by tick-borne disease infections and toxins. They have proven to increase the volume of the brain's gray matter, especially in areas that are responsible for regulating mood.

Omega-3 fatty acids come from both plant and animal sources. Ranges of 1,000–3,000 mg of eicosapentaenoic acid (EPA) and 1,000–1,500 mg of docosahexaenoic (DHA), when taken daily, have proven to significantly improve symptoms of depression, aggression, and other mental disorders, as well as protect against early cognitive decline and Alzheimer's disease.

Ken Singleton, MD, writes in his book *The Lyme Disease Solution* that many chronically ill people can't efficiently utilize omega-3 fatty acids from plant sources such as flax and hemp seed or walnuts. He instead recommends obtaining omega-3s from animal sources. Fish that contain low levels of mercury, such as salmon, herring, anchovies and sardines, are probably the best sources of omega-3 EFAs. Venison and free-range chicken, eggs, and beef also contain some omega-3 EFAs. Including these foods in the diet, along with a high-quality, low-mercury-containing fish oil product such as cod fish liver oil from Nordic Naturals, is important for healing neural tissue and thereby, depression.

Finally, the body can more easily absorb omega-3 fatty acids from food than from supplements. This is true of most nutrients, which is why supplements should never be used as a primary way of obtaining nutrition. Because our food supply is severely depleted in nutrients, however, and the nutritional needs of the chronically ill are much higher than those of the general population, supplements are nonetheless a necessary adjunct to a healthy diet.

Why Methylation Matters

Methylation is a somewhat complicated concept to understand, but I will try to provide a simple explanation here for the layperson. In short, methylation is a process in which certain chemicals, called methyl groups, are added to constituents of DNA, proteins, and other molecules, to keep them in good working condition. Methyl groups play a role in regulating gene expression, and enable all metabolic functions to take place in the body.

When a compound receives a methyl group, this initiates a reaction (such as turning on a gene that will silence a virus, or activating an enzyme). When the methyl group is lost or removed from the compound, the reaction stops (and the gene is turned off, or the enzyme is inactivated). Methylation processes regulate mood by "turning on" the production of serotonin and other neurotransmitters. If serotonin isn't methylated, it will become inactive, leading to depression. People who under-methylate have lower levels of serotonin than the general population. Methylation is also critical for the metabolism of catecholamines, the hormones produced by the adrenal glands in response to stress, which also play a role in mood regulation. Furthermore, melatonin, myelin basic protein, and CoQ10 synthesis are all dependent upon methylation processes, and also directly or indirectly influence mood. It is important to correct for any methylation defects, and provide the body with essential methyl donors, which aid in transferring methyl groups to other substances.

Tests for and Symptomatic Indicators of Methylation Defects

Here are some of the lab test results and symptomatic indicators that indicate methylation problems:

1. Having macrocytic anemia or large red blood cells

2. Having high homocysteine levels

3. Having inadequate methionine metabolism. Methionine is an amino acid that is converted to S-adenosyl methionine (SAM-e), the principal methyl donor for methylation of DNA, RNA, protein, phospholipids, creatine, and neurotransmitters. (Doctor's Data at www. doctorsdata.com and other reputable labs do methylation tests to measure different indicators of methionine metabolism).

4. Feeling unwell after taking amino acids

5. Responding well to SAM-e, zinc, or magnesium supplementation

Correcting Methylation Defects with Nutrients

S-adenosyl methionine (SAM-e) is one of the principal methyl donors involved in neurotransmitter synthesis and can be purchased as an over-the-counter supplement at health food stores. Trimethylglycine and creatine monohydrate are amino acids that increase SAM-e levels and may be a useful replacement for those who can't afford the more expensive SAM-e.

Folinic or 5-methyl-tetra-hydro-folate, zinc, B-vitamins, and especially methyl-B-12 also support methylation processes.

Vitamin B-12

Vitamin B-12 deficiencies are common in depressed people, as well as in those with Lyme disease. It's important to supplement for vitamin B-12 deficiencies, not only because vitamin B-12 plays an important role in methylation, but also because it protects against neurodegenerative diseases such as Parkinson's and Alzheimer's. Deficiencies of B-12 can cause irreversible neurological damage to the body.

Measuring Vitamin B-12 Levels in the Body

Unfortunately, standard lab tests that measure vitamin B-12 levels are unreliable and often give false high readings. The Centers for Disease Control (CDC), write on their website, www.cdc.gov, that homocysteine (Hcy) and methylmalonic acid (MMA) are the most common, accurate, and widely used confirmatory tests for identifying vitamin B-12 deficiencies. One of the website's authors also writes: "Because cobalamin is necessary for the synthesis of methionine from Hcy (homocysteine), low levels of vitamin B-12 lead to increases in total serum Hcy. The total serum Hcy test is a sensitive indicator for a vitamin B-12 deficiency."

Neurological and other symptoms can indicate a vitamin B-12 deficiency, as well, although it can be difficult to determine whether such symptoms are the direct result of a B-12 deficiency or some other cause. Symptoms of B-12 deficiency include:

- Mental confusion
- Delusions
- Paranoia
- Headaches
- Depression
- Pins and needles feeling in the extremities
- Balance problems
- A "buzzing" feeling in the body; tremors

The following gastrointestinal symptoms can also indicate B-12 deficiency:

- Nausea
- Vomiting
- Heartburn
- Bloating
- Appetite loss
- Weight Loss
- Diarrhea
- Constipation

Other symptoms of B-12 deficiency include:

- Fatigue (since B-12 is involved in red blood cell synthesis, and red blood cells transport oxygen to the other cells of the body)

- Paleness
- Shortness of breath that results from slight exertion
- White spots on the skin (typically the forearm) due to decreased mela-tonin production
- Pernicious anemia (because vitamin B-12 is involved in red blood cell synthesis)

Bioavailable Vitamin B-12 Supplementation

Studies have shown that oral forms of B-12 supplements aren't readily absorbed and utilized by the body, due to the complex metabolic pathways involved in B-12 metabolism. Hydroxy or methyl B-12 injections may be more effective, although these are only available by prescription. Cyano-cobalamin is rarely useful for people who are chronically ill, because most people with Lyme, chronic fatigue syndrome, and other severe health conditions cannot effectively convert it to methyl B-12, the more bioavailable form that the body requires (although paradoxically, it is the only form of injectable Vitamin B-12 available over-the-counter).

As a side note, when I went to a grocery store pharmacy in Denver, Colorado, to get a prescription for methyl B-12, the pharmacist told me that it was an expensive vitamin—around $1,000 for a 30-day supply of injections. I don't know if this is the standard cost among conventional pharmacies, but when I phoned a compounding pharmacy in Colorado, they told me it would cost less than $65 for a month's prescription of methyl B-12. Needless to say, I had my prescription filled at the compounding pharmacy. It pays to shop around for the best price on prescription nutrients and drugs.

If you can't afford B-12 injections, or don't have a doctor to prescribe them for you, Jarrow and Enzymatic Formulations are two sublingual brands of methyl B-12 which studies have shown to be useful for raising B-12 levels. They have also received high ratings from their users. Garry Gordon, MD, of Longevity Plus also makes a good product called Beyond B12, which contains methylcobalamin, along with three forms of folic acid, including 5-MTHF, a methylated form of folic acid.

Egg yolks, meat, liver, and oily fish are good food sources of vitamin B-12, although by themselves, are insufficient to reverse deficiencies. Dark, leafy green vegetables, sunflower seeds, wheat germ, fish, eggs, beans, walnuts, asparagus, almonds, and whole grains also support methylation.

The Importance of Eliminating Food Allergies

Food powerfully influences mood and mental function, and avoiding foods that cause or exacerbate inflammation is crucial for minimizing the severity of depression. Allergenic foods, for example, cause inflammation. Foods and substances that commonly produce an inflammatory response in people with chronic health problems include: wheat, alcohol, caffeine, potatoes, nightshade vegetables, gluten, eggs, peanuts, soy, corn, chocolate, cheese, tomatoes, dairy products, and even non-gluten grains. GMO (genetically modified) food also causes allergies, as do processed foods containing many additives and preservatives.

See Chapter Two for more information about what constitutes a healthy, non-inflammatory diet for people with chronic illness involving Lyme disease.

How Gut Health Influences Mood

The enteric nervous system, which controls the gastrointestinal (GI) tract, is comprised of tissue that lines the esophagus, stomach, small intestine, and colon. Eighty to ninety-five percent of the body's serotonin is produced here, along with other neurotransmitters. It is often referred to as the body's "second brain," since the health of the GI tract affects the brain, and vice versa.

William Whitehead, PhD, Professor of Medicine at the University of North Carolina, contends that the digestive system is closely attuned to a person's emotions and state of mind. People with irritable bowel syndrome often suffer GI symptoms during times of stress and anxiety. Even healthy people can have an increase of stomach pain, nausea, constipation, or diarrhea during stressful life events.

A constant exchange of chemicals and electrical messages occurs between the gut and the brain. Therefore, whatever affects the gut will directly affect the brain, and vice versa. Studies have found that gut health plays a key role in regulating mood and emotions.

According to Point Of Return, Inc. (www.pointofreturn.com), a nonprofit organization that was established to help people find freedom from dependence on sleeping pills, anti-anxiety medication, and antidepressants, a healthy lower intestine should contain at least 85 percent friendly bacteria to prevent over-colonization from harmful microorganisms. The body can remain healthy if it contains only fifteen percent bad bacteria. Unfortunately, most people have this balance inverted, and have much more harmful bacteria in their guts than beneficial.

Having an overgrowth of bad bacteria in the gut depresses immune function and reduces the production of enzymes that assist with nutrient absorption. Such nutrients are important for neurotransmitter synthesis. Bad bacteria also directly interfere with neurotransmitter production. It is vital to eliminate pathogenic bacteria from the gut and replace it with beneficial flora, in order to most effectively treat depression. More information about how to do this, as well as other aspects of GI health, is found in Chapter Seven.

Other Remedies for Depression

St. John's Wort is sometimes useful for healing depression because it contains hypericin, a substance that increases the concentration of serotonin in the central nervous system by inhibiting two enzymes responsible for its breakdown. Because this herb has been reported to increase anxiety in some people, those with anxiety may want to avoid it.

Balancing Estradiol and Progesterone

Low levels of estradiol (a type of estrogen) can also contribute to depression, especially in women, since estradiol increases the brain's ability to retain serotonin. Similarly, progesterone deficiencies can cause or contribute to depression. Progesterone and estrogen balance one another in the body, so a deficiency of one will lead to an excess of the other. Most women have low progesterone levels and PMS, perimenopausal and menopausal symptoms as a result of having too many harmful chemical contaminants in their bodies. This is because these chemicals mimic estrogen in the body. Too much of the wrong type of estrogen causes an imbalance in the estrogen-progesterone ratio, leading to depression and other symptoms. Most men also have excessive amounts of xenoestrogens, (as these "fake" estrogens are referred to). Phthalates, which are found in plastics, are one major source of xenoestrogens. They create hormonal imbalances that can cause or contribute to depression.

Healing from depression caused by low estrogen or low progesterone requires supplementing the body with bioidentical hormones or natural progesterone and estrogen products derived from plant sources (the latter of which can be obtained from most health food stores).

Pharmaceutical companies market harmful synthetic forms of progestins (they aren't called "progesterone" because they aren't really progesterone) and estrogens to women who have progesterone and estrogen deficiencies. Two of these products, Provera and Premarin, are chemically dissimilar to human hormones. Because of this, they create other problems in the body and increase women's risk for heart attacks, stroke, cancer, and other medical problems. The results of a 2002 Women's Health Initiative study in which 16,608 postmenopausal women, aged fifty to seventy-nine, were given either Provera or Premarin, revealed that these women had 41 percent more strokes, 29 percent more heart attacks, 26 percent more breast cancer, and a 76 percent increase in Alzheimer's dementia than women who were given placebo pills. These side effects didn't occur among women who used bioidentical hormones or natural, plant-derived products that support hormone production, because such products are chemically identical to what the body produces.

Other hormones, especially the adrenal hormone cortisol, as well as thyroid hormone, also powerfully influence mood. See Chapter One for more information about balancing these hormones.

In Summary

Emotional trauma and the depression that often results from such trauma may be the most common cause of immune suppression when immune suppression wasn't initially caused by pathogens or toxins. Healing the immune system in such cases requires more than just taking some vitamin C or immune-modulating herbs. It requires healing the source of trauma by learning to adopt healthier beliefs, thoughts, and behavioral patterns. These are tasks that, for some people, should be accorded at least as much attention as protocols for killing pathogens or removing toxins. It also requires restoring the biochemistry with mood-supportive nutrients and bioidentical hormones, which are often radically depleted by trauma, infections, and toxins.

Chapter Nine

Other Conditions That Contribute to Disease in People with Tick-Borne Infections

Other conditions cause illness in people with tick-borne infections. Some play a relatively minor role in the overall symptom picture, while others are primary causes of symptoms and disease. Regardless of their importance, treating them is essential for a full recovery from chronic illness. In the following sections, I briefly describe what some of these conditions are, along with treatments for each one. Not every cause of chronic illness is described here; just some of the most important ones, based on my research and experience. The information contained within the following sections is only meant to provide a broad overview of some of the other contributing factors to disease. It is not meant to be a comprehensive guide. Therefore, additional resources for exploring each topic will be recommended within, or at the end of, each section.

Other Causes of Chronic Illness in People with Tick-Borne Infections

- Candida (and other types of fungal overgrowth)
- Opportunistic viruses, bacteria, and other pathogens
- Foci infections in the mouth
- Structural problems
- Other environmental toxins and compromised detoxification mechanisms

Candida (and Other Types of Fungal Overgrowth)

Candida (candidiasis) and other types of systemic fungal overgrowth result when the immune system is weakened by toxins, prolonged antibiotic therapy, infectious organisms, and other stressors. Even people who maintain a near-impeccable diet, free of natural and artificial sugars, can be susceptible to developing yeast and other fungal infections when their immune systems aren't functioning properly.

Candida Symptoms

Common Candida (and other yeast infection) symptoms include, but aren't limited to:

- Chronic vaginal yeast infections
- Coated tongue
- Gastrointestinal dysfunction
- Bloating
- Chronic dermatitis
- Fatigue
- Chronic sinusitis
- Carbohydrate intolerance or allergies
- Cognitive dysfunction

Candida and Immune Suppression

Candida infections may reside only in the gastrointestinal tract, or they may be systemic. They can infect multiple organs and tissues, and may or may not respond to antifungal therapy. As Morton Teich, MD, noted at the 2011 International Lyme and Associated Diseases Society (ILADS) conference, some people are chronically sensitive (susceptible) to Candida, and only a subset of patients will respond well to dietary modifications and antifungal treatments. Some people with Lyme disease are unable to eliminate Candida as long as their immune function remains compromised by tick-borne infections and toxins, even if they do antifungal treatments and maintain a yeast- and sugar-free diet. This can be extremely frustrating for the afflicted, especially since anti-Candida diets are demanding and difficult for most people.

While Candida results from a weakened immune system, it also causes immune dysfunction. At ILADS, Dr. Teich noted that Candida causes an imbalance of pro- and anti-inflammatory cytokines and secretes substances that impair immune function. Healing the gut is therefore essential to healing from systemic Candida infections. This involves ridding the GI tract of not only Candida, but also other pathogenic organisms and the biofilms that reside there, and then replacing those pathogens with healthy bacteria by using probiotic supplements and fermented foods. See Chapter Seven for more information on healing the GI tract.

Candida Treatment

Many people with chronic Lyme disease also have Candida infections. Lyme-literate doctors have different approaches to treating these infections. Some doctors will treat their patients' Candida prior to commencing antibiotic or antimicrobial therapy. The rationale behind this approach is that by eliminating Candida first, the patient becomes less susceptible to yeast infections during antibiotic treatment and is better able to fight tick-borne infections, because one of the immune system's burdens has been removed.

While treating fungal infections at the outset of treatment may be beneficial for some people, prolonged antibiotic therapy tends to encourage Candida growth, regardless of the person's yeast infection status prior to starting antibiotics. Antibiotics remove beneficial bacteria from the body and create a hospitable environment in which Candida and other yeasts can easily flourish. Also, it may not be possible to fully eliminate Candida as long as tick-borne infections are helping to "hamstring" the immune system.

Other doctors treat their patients' fungal infections at the same time as the tick-borne infections. Such doctors believe that taking antifungal remedies during antibiotic therapy helps to keep Candida and other yeast overgrowth to a minimum. Nystatin, Diflucan, and a variety of natural remedies (some of which will be listed in the following paragraphs) are used for this purpose.

Still other doctors don't administer any antifungal therapy to their patients until after their patients finish their antibiotic treatments for tick-borne infections. They believe that the Candida and other yeast infections will simply continue to grow and flourish as long as they are on antibiotics, so it doesn't make sense to treat their fungal infections until the very end of treatment.

The second approach—treating tick-borne infections at the same time as Candida—makes the most sense to me. If patients aren't given antifungal remedies until after they finish their antibiotic therapy, by the end of their treatment they may have developed a massive systemic yeast infection. (This isn't true for those who use natural antimicrobial remedies to treat tick-borne infections. Unlike antibiotics, natural remedies don't eliminate healthy gut bacteria, which are the body's first line of defense against fungal and other types of infections). Widespread yeast infections may be difficult to treat and may compromise the immune system so that the body can't fully heal from Lyme and other problems. The body may be unable to eliminate all Candida as long as it is being given antibiotics, but concurrently administering antifungal treatments will help to keep the Candida in check until the antibiotic therapy is finished, at which time antifungal therapy should be continued until no symptoms of Candida remain.

Natural and Pharmaceutical Anti-Fungal Remedies

Diflucan and Nystatin are the most widely prescribed pharmaceutical medications for treating fungal infections. Diflucan is a better antifungal remedy for people with systemic yeast infections. Nystatin only eliminates infections in the gut. Nystatin may be a less desirable option because it contains sugar—an ironic addition to a drug that is supposed to eliminate sugar-induced yeast infections! Because sugar also feeds tick-borne infections, Nystatin may not be the best choice for people with Lyme disease.

Many natural remedies, especially when used in combination, can also be extremely effective for treating Candida and other fungal infections. Such remedies include:

- Oregano
- Caprylic acid
- Citrus seed extract
- Grapefruit seed extract

- Garlic
- Tea tree oil
- Colloidal gold
- Taheebo tea

Treating Candida and other yeasts using a one size fits all approach is usually ineffective, since people's biochemistries differ. I suffered from symptoms of Candida even prior to taking antibiotics for tick-borne infections, but was able to effectively treat it by eliminating certain foods from my diet and by taking thirty drops daily of TriGuard® Plus, a natural, inexpensive remedy comprised of grapefruit seed extract, colloidal gold, and tea tree oil.

Immune-boosting substances such as transfer factors, which are found in colostrum, may also be helpful for eliminating Candida. Researched Nutritionals (www.researchednutritionals.com) makes quality transfer factor products, although they are only available via prescription. 4Life Research USA (http://transferfactor-4-life.com) also makes good products, which some Lyme-literate health care practitioners use for boosting their patients' immune function.

The Importance of Maintaining an Anti-Candida Diet

To eliminate Candida and other yeast infections, it's usually not enough to only take antifungal remedies. It's also important to avoid certain foods, including most grains and grain products, fruit, sugars (natural and otherwise), peanuts (and other allergenic nuts), legumes, potatoes and other starchy vegetables, mushrooms, gluten, soy, corn, artificial sweeteners/additives/preservatives, alcohol, caffeine, and dairy. All of these foods encourage yeast growth. The Candida Diet website contains a comprehensive list of foods to avoid during Candida treatment (www.theCandidadiet.com/foodstoavoid.htm). Some people may need to follow a stricter diet than others.

Replenishing the body with probiotics is another important step in healing from Candida, since the bacteria found in probiotic foods and supplements help the immune system to combat yeast infections. Probiotics replenish beneficial bacteria, not only in the gut, but also the entire body. See Chapter Seven for more information on effective sources of probiotic foods and supplements.

Treating Candida is an important component to recovery from chronic illness involving Lyme disease. A complete Candida elimination protocol involves all of the following:

- Taking antifungal remedies, both pharmaceutical and natural. (I believe that natural remedies should always be tried first, especially when infections are only mild or moderately severe. Severe infections may require a prescription drug, but I recommend drugs as a last resort. All pharmaceutical medications have adverse effects upon the body).
- Healing the gut, by removing all pathogenic organisms and their biofilms; repairing injured gut tissue with aloe vera, slippery elm, and marshmallow root; removing allergenic foods from the diet, and replenishing gut flora with quality probiotic products.
- Removing all foods that feed fungal infections.
- Strengthening the immune system with colostrum and/or other immune-boosting substances.

For more information on Candida, I recommend studying The Candida Diet website, www.theCandidadiet.com, or *The Body Ecology Diet* by Donna Gates and Linda Schatz.

Opportunistic Viruses and Bacteria

It is commonly believed within the Lyme disease community that *Borrelia, Babesia, Bartonella*-like organisms, *Ehrlichia*, and *Mycoplasma* infections are usually the main instigators of symptoms in people with tick-borne infections. They are found in most everyone with chronic Lyme disease.

Other infections are also often present in people with tick-borne illness. These infections are sometimes referred to as "opportunistic" because they don't cause symptoms until one or more of the above-mentioned tick-borne infections suppress the immune system. Some of these infections may be eliminated by the immune system without any outside intervention as *Borrelia* and the other principal tick-borne infections are treated with antimicrobial remedies. Some may also require treatment with antimicrobial remedies.

Sometimes opportunistic infections can be a main cause of symptoms in people with chronic Lyme disease. Yet some Lyme-literate doctors whom I've interviewed contend that treatment for these infections, especially viruses such as Epstein-Barr, coxsackie, and herpes, is either relatively ineffective or has little impact upon symptoms until the more important tick-borne infections are addressed. It probably depends upon the person, the virulence of the infections, and their overall role in the disease picture. As with other conditions of chronic illness, it may be difficult to discern whether they are a principal cause of symptoms, especially if the symptoms that they produce strongly overlap with those of tick-borne infections. But for some people, opportunistic infections may be just as much of a problem as *Borrelia*, *Babesia*, and other common tick-borne infections.

Opportunistic infections tend to include viruses such as Epstein-Barr, coxsackie, chlamydia, cytomegalovirus, and herpes, and bacterial infections such as staph and strep. These infections produce symptoms that may emerge during the initial phases of illness, at the same time when symptoms from tick-borne infections appear, while the person is being treated for tick-borne infections, or even afterwards.

The aforementioned represent just a sampling of the opportunistic infections that are commonly identified in people with chronic Lyme disease. People may still have others for which tests do not yet exist. Every year, researchers discover (usually through unconventional testing methods) new species of pathogens. This makes it more difficult to sort out the true causes of illness and symptoms in people with chronic illness and Lyme disease. People with Lyme, as well as their doctors, may have an incomplete idea about which organisms are causing symptoms. Conventional tests don't exist for every type of infection and existing tests can produce inaccurate results, for multiple reasons. For instance, the immune system may not mount an antibody response to an infection; or a random urine, blood, or saliva sample may not contain the necessary antigen, or microbe DNA, needed to identify the pathogen or infection. Laboratory diagnostic guidelines are also often flawed and based on inaccurate information.

Opportunistic microbes, along with tick-borne organisms, may also be difficult to detect because they live in protective biofilm communities where the immune system can't "see" them. Biofilm is a mucopolysaccharide matrix that is created when infectious organisms attach to one another, and then to a substrate comprised of extracellular DNA and proteins. Biofilm are also comprised in part, of minerals. These bug "blankets" promote intermicrobial communication and protect microbes from the immune system and from antimicrobial treatments. Multiple species of organisms may live within a biofilm community and exchange intraspecies as well as interspecies DNA, thereby creating new species of microbes for which no diagnostic tests exist. This may further complicate treatments for opportunistic as well as tick-borne infections.

Today most Lyme-literate doctors recognize the importance of treating biofilms along with microbes. Breaking down biofilms exposes microbes to the immune system, thereby allowing the immune system to more effectively eliminate them. No definitive treatment for biofilms yet exists, as knowledge about them is still relatively scarce. However, some doctors and researchers have found effective ways to break down and eliminate them. For example, Susan Marra, MS, ND, in my book *Insights into Lyme Disease Treatment* notes that her patients respond to antimicrobial treatments better when she uses enzyme products such as Boluoke®, nattokinase, and Zyactinase™, along with substances such as N-acetyl-cysteine and lactoferrin, to degrade the microbes' biofilm.

One study presented at the 2011 International Lyme and Associated Diseases Society (ILADS) conference revealed that NutraMedix's herbal remedies Banderol and Samento, when combined, were effective at breaking down biofilms. They also destroyed both the active and cystic forms of *Borrelia*. Furthermore, these two products are thought to be more effective than either Tindamax or Flagyl for destroying *Borrelia* cysts. For more information on these products, visit BioNatus' Ecuadorian website: www.nutramedix.ec, or NutraMedix's US website: www.nutramedix.com.

Some doctors advocate not taking certain minerals during antimicrobial therapy, since the microbes use them to make biofilm. The immune system, however, requires minerals to function properly. Since the immune system is what ultimately defeats disease (with the help of antimicrobial treatments), I believe that it makes more sense to give the body what it needs to function properly, and to trust that in doing so, the body will be able to effectively eradicate the infections.

Treating Opportunistic Infections

Doctors sometimes prescribe antiviral herbs and drugs to their patients to treat opportunistic viruses. Valtrex is one common medication used for viruses, but the consensus among doctors whom I have interviewed seems to be that its effectiveness is limited in removing viral infections. This may be because the body is contending with other, more important infections and may not have the resources to battle viruses until these other infections are under control. For instance, mold, *Borrelia*, and *Babesia* are generally thought to be more important causes of symptoms for most people than opportunistic viruses. Treating the former infections first is important if the body is to effectively mount an immune response against the viruses.

Some doctors believe that it's important to treat viral infections at the same time as tick-borne infections because viral infections sometimes cause major symptoms. As previously mentioned, symptoms of these infections may crop up at the same time as symptoms of tick-borne infections. Or, they may appear later, after the tick-borne infections have been adequately treated and a clinical diagnosis has proven that the tick-borne infections are no longer causing problems for the body.

Antimicrobial herbs and antibiotics are usually the treatments of choice for opportunistic infections of all types. Many remedies that are used for *Borrelia* and co-infections are also effective for treating opportunistic infections. I won't describe all of the remedies that are used to treat those infections here, as the list of infections and their corresponding remedies is long and varied. The choice of remedy also depends upon the individual person's biochemistry. In general, I believe that botanical remedies are a better first line of treatment for infections than pharmaceutical drugs. In addition to being less toxic to the body, botanicals are multifaceted in their properties, and often attack infections via multiple pathways; for instance, by simultaneously stimulating immune function, thwarting the microbe's survival mechanisms, reducing inflammation, and providing nutritive substances that heal and nourish the body.

Some people eliminate microbes using electromagnetic frequency therapy such as Rife and biophoton machine therapy. I don't believe that enough research has been done, nor enough patient experience documented to establish their effectiveness for treating all types of opportunistic infections. Of course, that information may be forthcoming. Both Rife and biophoton therapy have proven to be effective for eradicating *Borrelia* infections, however. As with most antimicrobial therapies, they may need to be combined with other antimicrobial treatments.

For more information on opportunistic infections, I recommend studying the 2011 International Lyme and Associated Diseases Society DVD presentations, which can be purchased at: www.ilads.org.

Foci Infections in the Mouth

Foci infections are infections that start in a localized part of the body (in this case, the mouth), but which eventually cause disease in other parts of the body, due to the spread of the infections and toxins that they produce. Foci infections caused by root canals and cavitations were once completely ignored by holistic doctors, but they are now being widely recognized as significant contributing factors to chronic illnesses of all kinds—including cancer and heart disease, as well as various autoimmune diseases.

Dental amalgams, which contain high amounts of neurologically damaging mercury, also severely compromise immune function and cause illness. Because amalgams have already been discussed at length in many other books on holistic wellness, their dangers will not be described here. For more information on illness caused by amalgams, I recommend reading *Amalgam Illness: Diagnosis and Treatment* by Andrew Cutler, or *Uninformed Consent: The Hidden Dangers in Dental Care* by Hal Huggins, D.D.S.

A strong relationship exists between the health of the mouth and the health of the entire body. California dentist P. Vernon Erwin, D.D.S., illustrates this concept on his website www.drerwin.com, where he writes:

"The oral structures are directly connected with the sinuses and upper respiratory tract. They are connected by nerves, blood and lymph vessels and so on, through which information or material can be passed along to and from every cell in the body. There are numerous routes for bacteria and other pathogens to migrate from the friendly confines of the oral cavity to anywhere they please, infecting and causing disease and dysfunction in any number of organs, depending on the type of bacteria and the condition of the immune system and biological terrain—your body's internal environment, the state of which largely determines whether and how you'll get sick."

Cavitations

Cavitations, or holes in the jawbone, are created when a socket isn't thoroughly cleaned after a tooth extraction. The socket becomes a breeding ground for bacteria. These bacteria often cause major infections and decay in the bone. The infections then spread and cause disease throughout the body.

People are usually unaware that jawbone infections and the cavitations that result from them can cause serious health problems, for several reasons. First, cavitations are difficult to diagnose, since they reside beneath the gums and can't be detected through x-rays or by a visual inspection (although ultrasound imaging devices such as the Cavitat can detect them). Second, most dentists (even biological or holistically-minded ones) don't routinely test their patients for potential infection from root canals or from wisdom tooth and other types of tooth extractions. Third, cavitations may be the result of tooth extractions that were done many years ago, during childhood (remember having your teeth pulled?) and therefore seem to have no relevance to current symptoms. Finally, many people with cavitations have no pain in their mouths or in the jawbone area. Cavitations can cause head and neck pain, but many people don't correlate these symptoms with problems in the mouth.

Bob Jones is the inventor of the Cavitat device. He recovered from ALS after having surgery to remove foci infections that were caused by cavitations in his jawbone. He has studied several thousand wisdom teeth sites and found 94 percent of them to contain cavitations (and therefore, infections) of various sizes and severities. He has also found 100 percent of all root canals to be infected. These infected cavitations produce varying degrees of illness, and can even be a main cause of symptoms in people with Lyme and other diseases. I personally know several people who believe that cavitation surgery was at least as important for their recovery as doing antimicrobial treatments for tick-borne infections.

One of them is Perry Louis Fields, who, in her recently released book *The Tick Slayer,* describes how her infected cavitations (which resulted after she had her wisdom teeth removed) were a major cause of her symptoms. Her recovery process accelerated dramatically when she had these cavitations cleaned out. Reading her book, I had the impression that cavitation surgery produced the most radical positive changes to her well-being, more than any other treatment or therapy.

Unfortunately, at the present time, there is no good non-invasive way to heal the body of these infections and the cavitations that they cause. Most good biological dentists recommend surgical debridement, which involves scraping the infected area clean to remove all diseased bone and infection contained therein. This process is invasive and difficult and must be done properly, or infections can easily return to the area. Perry Fields's biological dentist, William P. Glaros, D.D.S., writes on his website www.biological-dentist.com:

> "... It is not sufficient to "punch" a small hole in the bone, drill a little and rinse it out. In fact, this, and the practice of injecting these lesions with homeopathics and other substances, may very well increase the severity of the lesion instead of lessening it. After the unhealthy bone is removed, the goal is bone regeneration. Up to this point in time, successful bone regeneration has relied a great deal on the healing capacity of the individual's body and the treatment or elimination of predisposing and risk factors, which is not always possible. Lack of healing or reoccurrence of a lesion and the need for retreatment is always a possibility, no matter how well the surgery is performed. There are very few dentists who are trained in effectively diagnosing and treating these lesions. Those who are not so trained are not qualified to diagnose this condition or confidently assure patients that they do not have cavitations."

Treating cavitations is not a matter to take lightly. The surgery can be difficult, and people with compromised immune systems (such as those with Lyme disease) may or may not fare well as a result of the surgical procedure. That said, because cavitations can cause severe illness in the body, people who have unsuccessfully tried everything to treat their symptoms, and/or who suspect that cavitations may be a problem for them, may want to consider this treatment. It is important to choose a biological dentist who thoroughly understands cavitations and who has a good track record of success with their patients.

Hal A. Huggins, DDS, provides excellent recommendations on his website www.hugginsappliedhealing.com, for those looking for a biological dentist. Dr. Huggins is world-renowned for his work in holistic dentistry and has developed safe, effective protocols for treating cavitations and autoimmune diseases caused by dental toxins, which are now used by dentists worldwide. More information on dental toxins and Dr. Huggins' treatment protocols, as well as practitioner recommendations, can also be found on his website.

Root Canals

As with wisdom tooth extractions, root canal procedures also create systemic infections in the body. Root canals are deep fillings that are placed when tooth decay has penetrated deeply into the tooth. During the root canal procedure, the tooth's nerves and blood vessels are destroyed, so that the tooth becomes essentially dead. Then a filling is placed where the tissue and decay used to be. Unfortunately, studies have proven that even the best root canals fail to remove all harmful bacteria from the tooth, even if dentists thoroughly clean and sterilize the tooth area after the root canal procedure. These bacteria then proliferate and cause infection throughout the body. Many holistically-minded or biological dentists believe that root canals can be the triggering cause for autoimmune diseases of all kinds.

The fact that root canals cause systemic disease was demonstrated long ago by the famous dentist and researcher Weston Price, D.D.S. (1870–1948). Dr. Price discovered that if he extracted a root canal tooth from a person with a particular illness and then sewed that tooth under the skin of a rabbit, the rabbit would almost always develop the same type of illness as the person from whom the tooth came. Similarly, the Mayo Clinic, in the early 1900s, described finding bacterial growth in root canals. When these bacteria were transferred to lab animals, they created the same diseases in the animals that the donor humans had—anywhere from *80 to 100 percent* of the time. Unfortunately, this research and the information that links root canal infections with systemic illness has mostly disappeared from mainstream medical publications, and possibly even been suppressed by the American Dental Association.

The non-profit Toxic Element Research Foundation (TERF) believes that it is no coincidence that in the United States root canals abound in most people with certain types of autoimmune diseases, including MS, Lou Gehrig's disease, and arthritis. One study found that 97 percent of people with cancer have root canals. Reversal of these diseases often occurs when, as part of a comprehensive treatment program, root canal teeth are extracted, and the affected area of the mouth is thoroughly cleaned out.

The only way to ensure that root canal procedures won't cause immune-devastating illness in the body is by simply not having them done. The only alternative to an existing root canal is to have the infected tooth extracted, which means that the natural tooth will be lost. After the tooth is extracted, some people may choose to receive an artificial tooth implant to replace the missing tooth. Tooth implants are generally metallic posts that are implanted into the jawbone. They mimic lost tooth roots, but having titanium metal put into the bone may present its own health risks, in addition to being an expensive and complicated procedure.

Other people may choose to not replace the missing tooth at all, which may cause the other teeth to shift and thereby create jawbone misalignment, periodontal disease in adjacent teeth, and other problems that could affect the health of the body. Obviously neither of these root canal alternatives is without risk and potential health consequences. But it may be better to risk such consequences than to have a root canal procedure done, or leave an infected root canal in the mouth. There may yet be other alternatives to getting a root canal that I have not mentioned here, which are worth exploring with a biological dentist.

Summary of Foci Infections

The health of the mouth is integral to the health of the body. For some people with chronic Lyme disease, foci infections in the mouth, which result mostly from cavitations in the jawbone caused by tooth extractions and root canals, are a major cause of illness. Treating these infections includes removing all infected bone and tissue, and is essential for a full recovery from chronic illness. Jawbone cavitations severely compromise immune function and perpetuate systemic illness.

Environmental Toxins and Compromised Detoxification Mechanisms

Having compromised detoxification mechanisms is another major contributing factor to illness in people with tick-borne infections. I believe that detoxification problems are more often a symptom of another problem, rather than a primary cause of disease. For instance, *Borrelia* compromises immune function and destroys enzymes involved in detoxification, as do toxins such as heavy metals. Some people have genetic defects that predispose them to difficulties with removing toxins, but toxins themselves can cause a breakdown in the body's detoxification mechanisms. People who cannot effectively eliminate environmental toxins or biotoxins from pathogenic organisms may have a more difficult time healing from chronic illness than people who don't have such problems. Because detoxification is a large topic and this book focuses on primary, or instigating, causes of chronic illness, I will not be describing in detail all of the different factors that compromise the body's ability to remove toxins. Suffice it to say that many people are sick today due to exposure to environmental toxins, which are causing severe chronic illness of all kinds, including cancer, chronic fatigue syndrome, fibromyalgia, neurological illnesses such as Alzheimer's, Parkinson's, autism, and other autoimmune diseases. Having too many toxins in the body can also preclude recovery from chronic Lyme disease.

Several types of toxins, including electromagnetic pollution, mercury, chemicals, hormones and antibiotics, which are found in the air, and food and water supply, have already been described in this book. However, many other types of environmental contaminants also harm the body and cause illness. Among these are radioactive substances; most of which are heavy metals such as uranium, strontium, plutonium and cesium. Nowadays, everyone is being exposed to high amounts of these metals, especially since the nuclear meltdown event at Fukushima in March, 2011. Warfare weaponry, such as nuclear and dirty bombs, also release massive amounts of radioactive substances into the atmosphere and cause DNA alterations and cellular dysfunction, and consequently, cancer and autoimmune disease. Radioactive iodine in the atmosphere is also a huge problem. According to Lee Cowden, MD, human beings require approximately 30 mg of iodine per day for proper white blood cell function and proper binding of steroidal hormones to cell receptors. If insufficient amounts of non-radioactive iodine aren't ingested by the body (such as through Lugol's iodine solution), then the body will take up radioactive iodine from the atmosphere to meet its needs. The radioactive iodine either kills the cells that it enters, or causes DNA mutations that lead to cancer. Thus, supplementing with iodine is crucial for protecting the body against radioactive iodine.

Solvents and other man-made toxins such as auto exhaust, benzene, xylene, toluene in paints, solvents in construction adhesives, formaldehyde in carpet and chemicals that are found in skin-care and household cleaning products also accumulate in the body over time. They can cause illness when their levels get too high.

People with tick-borne infections are particularly susceptible to the effects of these toxins, since infectious organisms compromise the body's ability to detoxify. Everyone nowadays is affected to some degree by environmental toxins, the symptomatic effects of which vary from person to person. As the amount of industrial chemicals, radioactive substances, and other environmental toxins in the air, water, food, personal care products and industry continues to increase, such toxins are likely to become an ever-more prevalent cause of chronic illness, perhaps even more so than tick-borne infections.

Removing environmental toxins requires a multifaceted approach that involves supporting the body's natural detoxification processes, along with taking toxin binders to address the different types of toxins that are present.

Following are some general detoxification guidelines. Because toxins and detoxification is such a broad subject, I also recommend reading books, attending conferences and studying websites that are devoted exclusively to the subject. I merely include a few guidelines here to provide a general idea about what is involved in detoxification.

First, it's important to support the detoxification organs, which include the kidneys, liver, gallbladder, skin and lymphatic system. Optimizing the use of each one of these organs prevents the liver and kidneys from becoming overburdened as a result of having to do most of the work of toxin removal. Exercise and infrared saunas remove toxins via sweating. Body brushing and rebounding on a mini-trampoline stimulate the drainage of toxins through the lymphatic system, and facilitate their removal from the body. Coffee enemas, liver-supportive herbs and herbal products such as milk thistle and Liv-52, and foods that support hepatic function, such as beets, carrots and cucumbers, aid the liver and gallbladder in toxin removal, as do B-vitamins. Many herbs and natural foods also support kidney detoxification; among these are parsley, uva-ursi leaf, marshmallow root, celery and pineapple. Doing modified vegetable juice fasting and colonics, drinking a lot of lemon water, and taking clay and Epsom salt baths are other strategies which facilitate toxin removal. Many other detoxification strategies exist, but those I've just mentioned, especially those which involve the use of natural remedies and exercise, are among the most effective and inexpensive.

Homeopathic drainage remedies can also significantly support the body's natural detoxification processes. Pekana and Heel make excellent remedies that stimulate and facilitate the removal of toxins through the lymphatic system, kidneys and liver. NutraMedix also produces a variety of effective homeopathic and herbal remedies for this purpose, including Burbur Detox, Parsley Detox, Pinella Brain and Nerve Cleanse, Trace Minerals Relax/Detox, Zeolite, and Zeolite-HP.

Additionally, according to Lee Cowden, MD, creatine monohydrate, molybdenum, zinc, trimethylglycine, 5-methyl-tetrahdro-folate, and Vitamins B-6 and B-12 can help people with genetic detoxification defects to process toxins.

In addition to supporting the body's detoxification processes, it is essential to take toxin binders on an ongoing basis, to remove toxins that have accumulated in the body over time and those which the body is continually exposed to from the environment. The type of binders that should be taken depends upon the specific toxins that need to be removed. It is not usually prudent to remove multiple types of toxins at once, since the overall body burden of toxins may be high and taking too many binders at once can overload the detoxification organs.

For instance, it might be a good idea to focus first upon mercury removal, and then proceed to lead. Some binders will remove many types of toxins. It is important to discern what dosage of a particular binder will not overload the body. Working with a knowledgeable holistic health care practitioner is usually the best way to determine this. In addition to the heavy metal binders described in Chapter Five, glutathione, zeolite, modified citrus pectin, apple pectin and chlorella also bind metals, but these substances are generally weaker binders than, for example, DMSA or DMPS. These binders are also effective for removing industrial contaminants.

Many substances also protect the body from the harmful effects of radiation. According to Joseph Mercola, MD, in his article, "This Vitamin Can Radically Reduce Damage from Radioactivity from Fukushima," Vitamin D3 neutralizes the effects of radiation. Vitamins C and D protect against DNA damage from radioactive particles, as do chlorella and spirulina. Potassium iodide and coconut oil help to protect the thyroid against radioactive damage, and washing vegetables in Chlorox removes radioactive particles from food.

Finally, dental amalgams contain high amounts of dangerous mercury which continually leaches from the teeth into the bloodstream. It is important to get all dental amalgams removed and replaced with composite fillings that are made from material that is compatible with the body's biochemistry. It is essential to see a biological dentist who is trained in safe amalgam removal and in testing the body for appropriate compatible composite fillings. Not taking proper precautions when removing mercury from the mouth can cause even greater amounts of mercury to be released into the body. Also, using inappropriate dental materials to replace the amalgam fillings can cause autoimmune reactions in the body. It's important to find a dentist who tests the body to determine the types of fillings that are most compatible with each individual person's biochemistry.

Another important way to minimize heavy metal toxicity is to never get a vaccination, of any kind. Many vaccines contain thimerosal, a preservative that is comprised of nearly 50 percent mercury, by weight. Vaccinations have been strongly linked to autism, Parkinson's, Alzheimer's, and other neurological illnesses. As the use of vaccines has increased, so has the rate of childhood autism. According to the Centers for Disease Control, the current rate of autism is 1 in 88 people, although some experts have estimated it to be as high as 1 in 40. In the 1970s, the rate of autism was 1 in 10,000. I personally know several people whose children became autistic after having received multiple vaccines, and who can trace the onset of their children's autism to vaccinations.

In Summary

Environmental toxins are a major or primary cause of chronic illness in people with tick-borne infections. Removing these toxins and supporting the body's detoxification processes is therefore essential for recovery. In general, it is best to do multiple detoxification strategies simultaneously, but it's also important to not overload the body by taking too many toxin binders at once or doing treatments that are too aggressive for the body. One effective detoxification protocol might involve taking homeopathic drainage remedies for the liver, kidneys and lymphatic system, along with a couple of toxin-binding agents. This could be followed by a far-infrared sauna session and/or rebounding on a trampoline, or taking a brisk walk outdoors. Detoxification strategies should be undertaken not only on a daily basis while chronically ill, but also for life. We are all exposed daily to a multitude of toxins and must be diligent to keep their levels low in order to remain healthy.

Structural Problems

Many people with Lyme disease have vertebral misalignments (subluxations), which cause pain in the soft tissues, as well as dysfunction in the organ systems. Organ function is linked to the body's structure and musculoskeletal function, and vice versa. Lyme-literate osteopath Shawn Naylor, DO, in an interview with me, stated that: "Vertebral dysfunction can negatively impact organ systems, especially those that are innervated at that level of the spine. So for instance, if the third thoracic vertebra is out of alignment, that might impair or diminish the quality of neurological input and output at the heart, which could predispose a person to heart palpitations. But I think that the reverse is more often true; that is, whenever I suspect organ dysfunction, and then I look at the (corresponding) segment of the spine, I see asymmetry or other evidence of musculoskeletal dysfunction such as tenderness or increased muscle tension."

Dr. Naylor acknowledges that a relationship exists between organ function and the body's structure. He believes that the organs may benefit when vertebral subluxations or misalignments are corrected. However, his experience has been that structural problems don't preclude healing from chronic illness and Lyme disease. Of course, correcting these problems may be tremendously beneficial for some people's healing, and can help to alleviate symptoms caused by Lyme and other conditions. For example, my publisher, Bryan Rosner, of BioMed Publishing Group, received chiropractic adjustments while healing from Lyme disease and discovered that these greatly reduced his neurological symptoms. Correcting vertebral misalignments can be an important component of healing from chronic illness involving Lyme disease.

When I asked Dr. Naylor why the skeleton becomes misaligned in people with chronic illness and Lyme disease, he responded that it's primarily because the autonomic nervous system (ANS), which plays a vital role in maintaining structure, has a finite amount of "bandwidth." According to Dr. Naylor, the body requires a great deal of "neurological data processing" from the ANS in order for it to just be able to stand and walk—never mind to maintain proper alignment and posture. The ANS micromanages the body's physiology at a cellular level. If its "bandwidth" is being used up to fight stressors such as Lyme infections, toxins, or a poor diet, then there isn't much left to lend to maintaining proper structural alignment.

In an email to me, Dr. Naylor wrote, "I never fully appreciated this (concept) until one day, a few years ago, when I ate an ice-cream cone, and it caused me to have sudden pain in my neck. I wasn't hunched over a textbook or stuck in a bad airplane seat. I just ate the wrong food and it caused my alignment to 'go out.' The conventional medical paradigm is too compartmentalized to make sense of this kind of phenomena, but both the osteopathic and chiropractic traditions emphasize the interconnectedness of bodily functions. And I believe that the 'ANS bandwidth' theory effectively illustrates this." Whenever the ANS has used up its "bandwidth," a person will also feel more pain or have problems in previously damaged ligaments or other soft tissues that have been weakened by Lyme or other factors such as accidents.

According to Dr. Naylor, it isn't just sub-optimal ANS output that causes misalignment. *Borrelia* organisms prefer to reside in soft tissue, where there is less blood flow and less immunity. They can damage the tissues directly, by invading them, or indirectly, by inciting the immune system to produce an inflammatory response in an attempt to eradicate them. Many Lyme disease patients complain of chronic pain at sites of previous injury, and contend that their injuries are slow to heal. And because *Borrelia* likes to target and settle in areas of tissue where damage has previously occurred, it may be more difficult for such damaged areas to heal, as long as infections are present to cause further damage and ANS function remains suboptimal.

To make matters worse, *Borrelia* damages nerves, which carry information from the autonomic nervous system to the rest of the body and vice versa. According to Dr. Naylor, this means that damaged nerves end up transmitting inaccurate information from the peripheral nervous system (the nerves and ganglia outside of the brain and spinal cord) back to the central nervous system (CNS). Such information might include where one bone is located in space relative to another, or how much tension or load the body's structure is under. Similarly, information sent from the central nervous system to the peripheral nervous system to correct problems with alignment, for example, may not arrive at the periphery in its intended or original form.

Also, according to Dr. Naylor, the ligaments sustain micro tears as a result of the normal, day-to-day wear and tear of living. A healthy body easily repairs these tears, but people with Lyme disease may not be able to repair them properly. Dr. Naylor likens the immune system in a person with Lyme disease to a maintenance crew working in a war zone. He says, "If you send a highway maintenance crew into a war zone, the quality of their workmanship will be lower than it would otherwise be. They may not even be able to keep up with ongoing damage." If people with Lyme disease end up suffering greater traumas, such as a sprained ankle or car accident injury involving more tearing of ligaments and tendon structures, these will not heal as well as those in the person who doesn't have Lyme or another chronic illness. Nerve damage causes slower repair of soft tissues, which in turn contributes to vertebral misalignments and pain.

Infections also create biotoxins that are toxic to nerve tissue. They trigger inflammatory responses that damage nerves. Dr. Naylor says that "People with Lyme disease have a frayed nervous system. I think of it like wires that have sustained damage to their protective coating. In nerves, this coating is called myelin, and if it's damaged by inflammation or toxins, the nerves that it's supposed to insulate may fire prematurely."

To restore nervous system and structural health, Dr. Naylor recommends supplementing the body with phosphatidyl-choline (Phos-Chol), a fatty acid that is the primary building block of all cell membranes, but which is especially important to myelin cells. These cells require much more Phos-Chol than other cells. Dr. Naylor also advocates gentle bodywork (manipulative therapy for the body) for managing structural/musculoskeletal problems. In my interview with him, he stated, "There are lots of styles of body work out there, and people should experiment with different practitioners to find those who can best help them. If you are a wrestler (with a big body), you might want someone to 'pop and crunch you' (as far as adjustments), but if you have Lyme disease, the body would probably perceive that as a micro trauma which it wouldn't heal well from. This could contribute to ligament laxity down the road. I'm not against high-velocity manipulation, but the majority of Lyme disease patients probably won't find lasting, long-term results from that. Gentler techniques like cranial sacral manipulation and indirect myofascial release tend to be better."

Dr. Naylor also advocates prolotherapy injections, which cause the body to form new ligament tissue (ligaments connect bone to bone in the body). Infectious organisms and inflammation destroy ligament tissue. Prolotherapy injections can help to replace and strengthen that tissue. In prolotherapy, a non-pharmaceutical irritant solution such as dextrose (a sugar), pumice, phenol glycerine, or cod liver oil extract is injected into the area where connective tissue has been damaged by infectious organisms, injury, toxins, and other factors. This creates an inflammatory response through which fibroblasts (cells from which collagen and other connective tissue is made) are stimulated to produce new tissue. The end result is the formation of new ligament tissue, which promotes proper structural alignment and neuromusculoskeletal health.

Prolotherapy is a difficult technique to do well, because the location of the injections must be determined precisely; otherwise, it will be relatively ineffective. When done properly, however, prolotherapy is a safe, non-toxic technique that can improve pain symptoms by up to 80 percent. Dr. Naylor notes that practitioners are increasingly using "prolozone," a type of prolotherapy that involves injecting ozone gas into the tissue, instead of traditionally used substances such as dextrose and pumice. He says, "Like other prolotherapy practitioners who have started adding ozone to their injections, I'm achieving greater success (with my patients) with fewer treatments. They also experience less pain during the procedure. There is less need for precision, so the procedure is less technically difficult and can be done in less time (than traditional prolotherapy treatments)."

Dr. Naylor believes, however, that it's best for *Borrelia* and other Lyme disease–related infections to be in remission, or at least under control, before attempting prolotherapy. He contends that joint pain often diminishes with antimicrobial treatment and that treating infections may in of itself render injections unnecessary. For this reason, he's reluctant to "pull out the prolotherapy needles" if his patients are in an early stage of treatment for infections. Dr. Naylor also believes that it's important to remove as many stressors as possible from the ANS, to help the body to maintain proper structure. This includes removing toxins, infections, dental amalgams, and anything else that stresses the body, such as electromagnetic fields.

I believe that supporting adrenal gland health is also important. Adrenal function is tied closely to ANS function. I have observed that people with weak adrenal glands tend to be hypermobile. Hypermobility is a condition in which the joints stretch further than normal and which tends to promote vertebral subluxations. TMJ is also commonly found in hypermobile people. Having TMJ can cause lymphatic drainage obstruction and prevent toxins from leaving the body. Treating the adrenal glands may be helpful for restoring ANS function and consequently, structural integrity and neuromusculoskeletal health.

My Story of Healing from Musculoskeletal Problems

I have observed that treating musculoskeletal problems can be tricky. Lyme disease sufferers tend to not hold chiropractic or osteopathic adjustments of the spine very well. As Dr. Naylor mentioned, such adjustments may even be perceived by the body as traumatic. Throughout my healing journey, I have found chiropractic or osteopathic adjustments to be moderately helpful whenever my spine would become badly misaligned. I also found that they weren't effective (and even made me worse!) if I did them too often.

I have also learned that gentle adjustments tend to work better than aggressive ones. Aggressive adjustments sometimes cause more pain in chronically ill people. When correcting spinal misalignments (or vertebral subluxations), it's important to find practitioners who understand the unique needs of people with tick-borne infections and other chronic health conditions. Chiropractic or osteopathic manipulation can make symptoms worse if done improperly. For some people, it may not even be a good treatment option.

Some practitioners advocate yoga for people with Lyme disease, but I found that the twisting and other movements (such as sitting Indian-style on the floor) involved in yoga caused me to become even more misaligned. People who are hypermobile can become easily misaligned by doing yoga. I therefore don't recommend it for people with Lyme disease.

The type of body conditioning routine that was most helpful for me for maintaining proper structure was Pilates, which involves exercises that build muscle strength and endurance, especially in the "core" (the upper and lower abdomen and back). Pilates exercises involve the use of both mind and body. They are based upon the assumption that the mind can control the muscles, which is why both physical movements and mental imagery are important in the routines. Pilates exercises align the spine and pelvis, and encourage oxygen flow to the tissues. They improve coordination and balance, which is important for people with Lyme disease, who tend to have balance problems. It's important to work with a physical therapist or Pilates instructor who understands structural problems. Many good instructors are physical therapists. A proficient instructor can tailor a Pilates routine to your needs. One particular Pilates routine may help one person, but harm another.

Like Dr. Naylor, another treatment that I have found to be very helpful for restoring proper alignment, or symmetry to the spine, and for eliminating the pain caused by subluxations, is prolotherapy. Prior to receiving prolotherapy injections, I had suffered from extreme pain in my lower back and hip. I had so much hypermobility in my pelvic region that I had to wear a sacroiliac (SI) belt, just to keep my hips and pelvis aligned. Even with the belt, I still had terrible pain. After approximately eight sets of prolotherapy injections, in which I received anywhere from three to six injections over a period of a year, my pain diminished by about 60 percent and I no longer needed to wear the SI belt. Prolotherapy injections didn't cure me of lower back and hip pain but they helped to make my life tolerable again. I still can't sit for more than an hour on a soft chair or sofa, and I must maintain proper posture to avoid being in pain, but I feel much better than before.

The downsides of prolotherapy are: 1) at approximately 100–150 dollars per injection, it is an expensive therapy (and usually not covered by insurance); 2) creating new ligament tissue stresses the adrenal glands. I had to sleep ten hours for about five consecutive nights following the injections, and was more tired than usual during the day; and 3) Pilates or other core-strengthening exercises must be employed in conjunction with the injections, or the ligaments will simply become weak again, and the injections won't provide much benefit over the long run.

It can be difficult to discern the true source of back/hip/pelvic pain in people with Lyme disease, which means that prolotherapy may not help everyone. Some people hurt because the myelin sheath that covers their nerves has been destroyed by tick-borne infections. Others have magnesium deficiencies, or inflammation from other causes. Prolotherapy works best on people who have ligament and other connective tissue (e.g., tendon) damage from infections, injury, or repetitive stress. It is also an excellent therapy for those with ligament laxity and hypermobility.

Yamuna body rolling (www.yamunabodyrolling.com) is another activity that I have found to be moderately helpful for maintaining proper structure and nervous system function, as well as for reducing pain. Body rolling involves doing exercises on a small ball. These exercises elongate, loosen, and tone muscles, as well as increase the joints' range of motion. The exercises promote proper alignment and can leave you feeling as though you have just been given a light chiropractic adjustment. Yamuna Zake, the founder of Yamuna body rolling, says that the exercises "re-educate muscles to move more effortlessly, painlessly and logically."

Yamuna body rolling is an inexpensive option for those who can't afford Pilates classes or prolotherapy injections. It is probably the most effective at-home therapy I have found, aside from Pilates. That said, it's important to keep in mind that what is helpful for one person may not be for another, and people with Lyme disease may find other therapies, such as cranial-sacral therapy or acupuncture, to be more beneficial for treating musculoskeletal pain.

In Summary

The conditions mentioned in this chapter often cause symptoms and disease in people with tick-borne infections. In some cases, they are a primary cause of illness. These conditions include Candida (and other yeast infections), musculoskeletal problems, opportunistic and foci infections, environmental toxicity, and compromised detoxification mechanisms. Foci infections, especially, are thought to be a major trigger for some severe degenerative and autoimmune diseases, including Lyme. Regardless of their role in disease, it is best to treat as many of these conditions as possible, in order to achieve a full recovery from chronic illness.

Concluding Remarks

While not every major cause of chronic illness in people who have Lyme disease has been discussed in this book, I have attempted to describe, on a basic level, some of the most common and insidious underlying causes of disease. I hope that by now, you realize that "it's not all about Lyme disease" (if you didn't before!) and that other factors frequently cause illness in people with tick-borne infections. These factors are sometimes more important than the infections. While it may seem overwhelming to have to treat multiple causes of illness, knowing what's making people sick can empower you, the patient or practitioner, to find new strategies for healing when treating tick-borne infections has proven to be insufficient.

It is my hope that this work will spare you, the patient or person with health challenges, many months or years of unnecessary suffering and treatments, and open new doors to wellness. And it is my hope that you, the Lyme-literate or holistic healthcare practitioner, will gain new insights into what is really making people with Lyme disease so sick. Because for some of us, "It's not all about the bugs."

Appendix I

Information and Tips on Diagnosing and Treating Tick-Borne Infections

Disclaimer:

These are my personal notes from recent International Lyme and Associated Diseases Society (ILADS) conferences, as well as other Lyme disease–related conferences. I don't claim the information in these notes to be 100 percent accurate or comprehensive, as it was taken mostly from lectures rather than published material, correspondence, or recorded interviews. While I have attempted to accurately represent the information, I may have made mistakes in its interpretation. Please bear this in mind as you read.

For complete information on how to treat Lyme disease (*Borrelia*) and other tick-borne infections according to Lyme-literate doctors, refer to my book, *Insights into Lyme Disease Treatment: 13 Lyme-Literate Doctors Share Their Healing Strategies*, or the book by Ken Singleton, MD, *The Lyme Disease Solution*. Joseph Burrascano, MD, has also provided extensive Lyme disease treatment guidelines, which can be accessed at: www.ilads.org/lyme_disease/B_guidelines_12_17_08.pdf. Also, Stephen Harrod Buhner's book, *Healing Lyme* provides excellent information on how to treat Lyme using herbal remedies, as does Lee Cowden, MD, in my book *Insights into Lyme Disease Treatment* and on the NutraMedix website, www.nutramedix.com.

For people who wish to treat Lyme disease using electromedicine, Bryan Rosner's book *Lyme Disease and Rife Machines*, provides comprehensive information on how to do this.

Finally, James Schaller, MD, has written books on *Babesia* and *Bartonella* that provide in-depth information on how to treat these two serious tick-borne infections. For more information on these, as well as Dr. Schaller's other books, visit: www.personalconsult.com. A comprehensive *Babesia* and *Bartonella* symptom checklist that was compiled by Dr. Schaller is included in Appendix II of this book.

General Information about Tick-Borne Infections

- More than twenty species of the *Borrelia* spirochete infect humans, not just *Borrelia burgdorferi*. Many new varieties and genospecies of *Borrelia* have arisen in recent years due to the organism adapting to its local environment.

- *Borrelia* and other tick-borne pathogens, such as *Babesia* and *Bartonella*, are transmitted principally through the bite of a tick. The infection rate in tick populations varies by location and from year to year.

- There are many new emerging species of tick-borne infections. Tests do not exist for all of these pathogens.

- It is a myth that Lyme disease exists mostly in the northeastern United States. The Centers for Disease Control reports high numbers of Lyme disease in every state.

- *Borrelia* is able to evade the immune system via various mechanisms. For instance, it hides deep within tissues, within collagen bundles, and produces biofilm.

- Only 17 percent of people with Lyme disease recall ever having had a tick bite, and only 36 percent recall ever having had a rash that might be linked to Lyme.

- The number of actual organisms implicated in chronic Lyme disease is few, but they secrete high amounts of glycoproteins, lipids, and DNA, all of which are toxic or immune-suppressive. Chronic Lyme disease is a cytokine (inflammatory) and toxin illness perpetuated by persistent infection.

- Inflammation causes most of the symptoms found in people with Lyme disease. If you lower the inflammation in the body, it's possible to become symptom-free from Lyme, even if tick-borne microbes are still present.

- Infections may either suppress or stimulate the immune system, which in turn causes hormonal problems and autonomic nervous system dysfunction.
- Co-infections exist in nearly everyone with chronic Lyme disease. Nobody is infected with just the *Borrelia* organism. Many co-infections persist in the body despite long-term antimicrobial treatments to remove them.
- Being co-infected with the parasite *Babesia* worsens the immune dysfunction that *Borrelia* causes, increases damage to the tissues and organs, and renders *Borrelia* and other infections more treatment-resistant.
- The longer that a person is ill from Lyme disease, the more systemic dysfunction and organ and tissue damage occur.
- Allergies to food, drugs, and chemicals in the environment are common in people with Lyme.
- Many species of *Borrelia* exist, all of which share their genetic material with one another and alter their DNA on a regular basis.
- Chronic Lyme disease is a symptom complex of many co-infections, not just *Borrelia. Anaplasma, Ehrlichia, Babesia, Bartonella, Mycoplasma, Rikettsia*, and viruses are infectious organisms that are all now commonly found in ticks.
- Many tick-borne infections can be transmitted via the placenta and sexually, as well as through blood transfusions and bodily fluids.

Physiological Abnormalities Found in People with Chronic Lyme Disease

Lyme-literate doctor, Richard Horowitz, MD, believes that people with Lyme disease have many problems, not just tick-borne infections. A more appropriate term to describe their condition, according to Dr. Horowitz, is Multiple Chronic Infectious Disease Syndrome (MCIDS). All of the following should be considered in people with MCIDS:

1. Bacterial, parasitic, viral, and fungal infections/diseases, including (but not limited to) all of the following: *Borrelia,* ehrlichiosis/anaplasmosis, *Bartonella, Mycoplasma, Chlamydia*, RMSF, typhus,

Q-fever, *Brucella*, tularemia, *Babesia*, piroplasms, filiariasis, amebiasis, giardiasis, strongyloides, pinworm, EBV, HHV-6, HHV-8, CMV, St. Louis encephalitis, West Nile and XMRV virus, Powassan encephalitis, and other viral encephalopathies.

2. Immune dysfunction

3. Inflammation

4. Toxicity

5. Food, drug, environmental, and other allergies

6. Nutritional and enzyme deficiencies

7. Mitochondrial dysfunction

8. Psychological stress

9. Endocrine abnormalities

10. Sleep problems

11. Autonomic nervous system dysfunction

12. Gastrointestinal problems

13. Drug use/addictions

14. Deconditioning (lack of exercise)

Note: Dr. Horowitz will be publishing a book in 2013 that addresses all of these conditions, and treatments for each.

- People with Lyme disease have a number of physiological problems, including disruption of the hypothalamic-pituitary-adrenal axis and the endocrine system; insulin resistance, autonomic nervous system dysfunction, blood vessel inflammation (which causes circulation problems), metabolic and mitochondrial dysfunction, and detoxification defects that prevent them from eliminating *Borrelia* and other pathogenic toxins, as well as environmental toxins.
- Lyme disease affects every part of the nervous system. Neuropsychiatric symptoms of Lyme disease may cause problems such as depression, extreme irritability, anxiety, paranoia, dementia, schizophrenia, bi-polar and obsessive-compulsive disorders, and anorexia nervosa.
- Lyme disease may mimic other illnesses. Symptoms may be similar

to those found in arthritis, chronic fatigue syndrome, fibromyalgia, Parkinson's, Lupus, ALS, multiple chemical sensitivity disorder (MCS), and multiple sclerosis, among others.

Diagnosing Lyme Disease

- Lyme should always be diagnosed clinically; that is, based upon signs and symptoms of illness, in addition to employing tests for infections and other tests that can indirectly indicate the presence of infections.

- Test results are often inaccurate. Most physicians are not taught how to properly identify chronic Lyme disease based upon symptoms. The official position of the Centers for Disease Control is that the disease does not exist. For these reasons, it is common for people to be improperly diagnosed or diagnosed many months or years after being infected. People with neuropsychiatric symptoms of Lyme are diagnosed, on average, two years after the onset of symptoms.

- To properly diagnose Lyme disease, healthcare practitioners must consider all of the following: 1) the patient's potential exposure to ticks and their personal history, including where they have worked, traveled, and spent recreational time; 2) the patient's symptoms (a complete list of Lyme disease symptoms, based on Dr. Joseph Burrascano's work, is available in the online document "Advanced Topics in Lyme Disease: *Diagnostic Hints and Treatment Guidelines* for Lyme and Other Tick Borne Illnesses" at www.lymenet. org/BurrGuide200810.pdf); 3) test results for specific infections as well as results from other types of tests that may indirectly indicate Lyme (i.e., the CD-57 and those that measure various inflammatory markers), and 4) whether the patient might have other illnesses, in addition to Lyme disease, or an illness that presents with similar symptoms to those found in Lyme disease.

- Lyme-literate health care practitioners should not assume that all of their patients' symptoms are due to Lyme disease. There may be other problems in the body that are causing symptoms.

- People with *Borrelia* infections have symptoms that "flare" every four weeks, according to the life cycle of the organism. These symptoms also tend to be migratory and change over time.

- Over eighty co-infections may be implicated in chronic Lyme disease, but it isn't necessary to test for all of these infections, since there are only so many medications that can be given to eliminate them. (So chances are, medications that work for some of the testable co-infections, will work for others that haven't, or can't, be tested for).

Borrelia Symptoms

- Common *Borrelia* symptoms include, but aren't limited to: fatigue and headaches; muscle, joint, and neuropathic pain (the latter is caused when the nerves of the peripheral nervous system, or that which is outside of the brain and spinal cord, are damaged); vision problems, insomnia, attention deficit disorders, speech problems, cognitive dysfunction, memory loss, and difficulty reasoning; mood disorders including depression, rage, and anxiety; orthostatis (blood pressure that drops upon standing), low libido, gastrointestinal dysfunction, weight gain or loss, light and sound sensitivity; stiff, sore muscles, and food sensitivities.
- Symptoms can change over time and worsen due to stress, the menstrual cycle, co-morbid conditions, and other factors.
- Symptoms tend to manifest initially and predominantly in the musculoskeletal, peripheral, and central nervous systems, as well as the heart. As the illness progresses, more body systems and organs become affected.
- According to some doctors, late-stage symptoms of *Borrelia* can develop over months or years. Arthritis-like symptoms may appear first, and develop less than six months following a tick bite. Central nervous system and peripheral nervous system symptoms may develop approximately 1–2 years following infection.

Lab Tests for Borrelia

- The enzyme-linked immunosorbent *assay* (ELISA) test has typically been recommended by the IDSA (Infectious Diseases Society of America) and CDC (Centers for Disease Control) to test for *Borrelia*, but many people with Lyme test negative for *Borrelia* with this test. Paradoxically, the sicker the person is, the greater the possibility that he or she will test negative for *Borrelia* using ELISA.

- The Western Blot test is another commonly recommended way to test for *Borrelia*. Its sensitivity is somewhat higher than that of the ELISA. About half of the people with *Borrelia* infections will test positive for infections using this test. As with the ELISA test, the more ill a person is, the less likely he or she is to test positive with this test. IgeneX, Inc. (www.IgeneX.com) provides the most accurate Western Blot test results in the United States, and possibly worldwide.

- People may have false-negative Western Blot test results if: 1) *Borrelia* is hiding in their cells in cystic form; 2) they have a suppressed antibody response; 3) the antibodies to *Borrelia* are hiding within immune complexes; or 4) *Borrelia* levels in the body are too low to create an immune response. Other reasons for a negative Western Blot test also exist.

- PCR (polymerase chain reaction) tests have a lower sensitivity to *Borrelia* than the Western Blot test, and can detect *Borrelia* approximately 30 percent of the time. Sensitivity to this test can be increased by taking antibiotics for a few days prior to testing. For best results, several test samples should also be collected. The CDC, as well as most insurance companies, do not accept PCR results as proof of infection.

- A new test, called the urine antigen capture test, detects *Borrelia* DNA in the urine. The only problem with this type of test (as with others that look for the DNA of an organism) is that because bacteria aren't uniformly present in body tissues or fluids, false-negative test results are common. Like the PCR test, sensitivity to this test may be increased by taking antibiotics for several days prior to testing.

- Another new test, called the T-cell stimulation assay, may also be useful for detecting *Borrelia* infections. It looks for the presence of proteins from *Borrelia* within certain immune system cells, such as T-cells. As with all tests, however, it has its limitations. Not everyone with *Borrelia* tests positive to infection. This test may also only reflect a person's exposure to the *Borrelia* organism, rather than their current infection status.

- Finally, another new promising type of test involves culturing *Borrelia* in the laboratory. Typically, this has been difficult to do, but new methods are now making it easier. Because culturing is a direct way to measure the presence of live organisms within a tissue sample, sensitivity to culture testing could be as high as 80 percent, according to some estimates. People with *Borrelia* who would ordinarily test negative to the infection on another type of test would be likely to test positive via culture testing. *Advanced Lab Services*, www.advanced-lab.com, now offers this test for *Borrelia*. (Another benefit to culture testing is that all species of *Borrelia* that a person is infected with can be tested for. Currently, most labs can only detect a few species of the organism, but more than twenty are known to infect humans.)

- Spiro Stat Technologies offers PCR-type testing for a large number of tick-borne infections, including multiple species of *Borrelia*. David Snow, PhD, associate director of Spiro Stat, describes the testing as a two-component process. In an email to me, he explained this process: "In the first component (of testing), the non-host (non-human) genetic material in the sample is amplified using a PCR-based technology. In the second component, the amplified genetic material is sequenced. The sequence information is then compared to the genomic sequences of all known insect vector-borne pathogens. The power of this technology allows Spiro Stat to detect and identify virtually all insect vector-borne pathogens in a single sample at the same time, without doing multiple test assays. This drastically reduces the cost (of testing) to the patient. There is no question that sequencing is the most accurate method of identification possible, since the genomic sequence is what defines an organism."

- The C4a test may indirectly indicate the presence of *Borrelia*, as levels tend to be elevated in people with *Borrelia* infections. The degree of elevation correlates with the severity of illness. If treatments are working, C4a levels should progressively decrease. (C4a is an inflammatory marker test).

- CD-57 scores sometimes indicate the severity of Lyme disease. A number that is less than 20 may indicate severe illness, and that the person is also co-infected with *Mycoplasma*. When CD-57 numbers are above 60, it indicates that *Borrelia* activity in the body is minimal. (Results of the CD-57 test aren't valid for determining the severity of *Borrelia* in children).

Treating Borrelia

- Doctors treat *Borrelia* in different ways. At one extreme, they may administer multiple high doses of toxic antibiotics at the outset of treatment. At the other extreme, they may start their patients off on low doses of just one or two moderately toxic antibiotics, and gradually ramp up the dosage and/or number and type of drugs over time. The advantage of the more aggressive approach is that it reduces the risk of microbes becoming resistant to pharmaceutical or herbal regimens. However, higher doses of very toxic remedies can cause more problems and side effects in the body. A more gentle approach causes less harm to the body, but infections may become resistant to less aggressive treatment regimens.

- Some doctors advocate pulsing treatments for *Borrelia*; for example, doing treatments for four days on, three days off. The advantage to pulsing treatments is that people can usually tolerate more aggressive regimens when treatments are administered with a break in-between. Pulsing can be used for most types of *Borrelia* medications. (Pulsing doesn't work for all tick-borne infections, especially *Babesia*).

- *Borrelia* exists in three forms: 1) as a spiral-shaped bacteria that has a cell wall; 2) as an L-shaped (or spiroplast) bacteria that lacks a cell wall; and 3) as a cyst that resides dormant in the tissues. Different medications/remedies must be used for each form of the organism, and these remedies must work both on the inside and outside of the cell. Multiple combinations of different types of antibiotics must be used for maximum effectiveness. According to Lyme-literate doctors, these include: 1) cell-wall drugs for the spirochete, or spiral form of *Borrelia* (penicillins such as amoxicillin and bicillin; cephalosporins such as Ceftin, Omnicef, IV Rocephin, and IV Claforan, and IV vancomycin or Primaxin); 2) tetracycline and erythromycin drugs (such as doxycycline and minocycline) for the L-form (spiroplast) of *Borrelia;* and 3) metronidazole, tinidazole, tigecycline, and rifampin for the cystic form. Macrolides, such as azithromycin and biaxin, and quinolones (such as Ciproflaxin and Levaquin) are useful for treating intracellular forms of the organism.

- Some Lyme-literate doctors believe that the choice of whether to use oral or intravenous antibiotics should depend upon various factors, including: 1) the age and physical constitution of the patient (people with weaker constitutions may not tolerate intravenous antibiotics); 2) the severity of disease and whether the patient has had symptoms for longer than a year; 3) whether the patient has acute carditis (inflammation of the inner tissue of the heart), 4) whether the patient has a high white blood cell count, 5) whether the patient is severely immunocompromised and/or has been on steroids, and 6) whether the patient has already failed oral antibiotic therapy.

- Intravenous antibiotic therapy must be given for a minimum of six weeks. (Specific examples of effective IV and oral antibiotic regimens, according to Joseph Burrascano, MD and Richard Horowitz, MD are found on the 2011 ILADS conference slides, which can be purchased at the following ILADS link: http://ilads.org/ilads_media/lyme-disease-videos-home).

- Herbal remedies can be used as standalone treatments for *Borrelia* and other tick-borne infections, or as a complement to antibiotic therapy. Herbs can, in some cases, be just as effective as antibiotics for treating infections, if not more so. For example, in vitro, Nutra-Medix's herbal remedies Banderol and Samento totally dissolved biofilms and rendered *Borrelia* more susceptible to antibiotics. Combined, they were also found to be more effective for eliminating cysts than all types of cyst-busting antibiotics.

- In addition to metronidazole and tinidazole, tigecycline may be useful for treating the cystic form of *Borrelia*. Some Lyme-literate doctors believe metronidazole to be the most effective drug for removing cysts, although it tends to produce the most side effects of all of the cyst-busting drugs.

- Treatment regimens for *Borrelia* (as with regimens for other tick-borne infections) must be rotated and modified on a regular basis, since the organisms quickly adapt to antibiotic and herbal remedies. Doctors may rotate their patients' regimens on a monthly basis, every six weeks, or every several months.

- Chronic tick-borne infections that have been present in the body for longer than six months usually require treatment for anywhere from six months to several years, and sometimes, indefinitely. The average treatment time is two to three years.

Bartonella Symptoms

Symptoms of *Bartonella* infection include, but are not limited to: insomnia, fatigue, arthralgia, dizziness, headache, seizures, memory loss, myalgia (muscle pain), depression, psychiatric symptoms (especially anxiety), bowel discomfort, muscle weakness and twitches, irritability, odd rashes, and eye pain. (For a more comprehensive list of *Bartonella* signs and symptoms, see notes from James Schaller, MD, in Appendix II).

Lab Tests for Bartonella

- Polymerase chain reaction (PCR) and antigen tests can be used to test for two species of *Bartonella*: *Quintana* and *B. henselae*. Neither of these tests, however, should be relied upon to definitively diagnose the infection. False-negative test results are common, and many other species of *Bartonella* exist for which tests have not yet been developed. Clongen, Medical Diagnostics Laboratory, and IgeneX may have the most useful lab tests for diagnosing *Bartonella*.
- A *Bartonella* diagnosis should be based primarily upon symptoms, and can be confirmed through a variety of bioenergetic testing devices such as the ASYRA or ZYTO, which detect the energetic frequencies of different organisms.

Treating Bartonella

- To effectively treat *Bartonella* with pharmaceutical medications, it is usually necessary to take two drugs, such as doxycycline and rifampin. Levaquin is also used but has been associated with undesirable side effects, and so may be better used as a last resort.
- Many herbal remedies are also effective for treating *Bartonella*, including NutraMedix's Samento, Banderol, and Cumanda. Clove bud oil and Houttuynia are also used by some practitioners.

Babesia Symptoms

Babesia symptoms include, but aren't limited to: chills, flushing, day or night sweats, fatigue, joint pain, cognitive dysfunction, headaches, and depression. (For a more comprehensive list of *Babesia* signs and symptoms, see notes from James Schaller, MD, in Appendix II.)

Lab Tests for Babesia

- As with *Bartonella*, PCR and antibody tests may be used to detect *Babesia*, but results from these tests are often inaccurate. Another test, the fluorescent in situ hybridization test (FISH), detects the presence of *Babesia* RNA (genetic material) through blood samples, but also has a high false-negative detection rate. One advantage of the FISH test, however, is that unlike other types of lab tests, it can detect other species of *Babesia* in addition to *Babesia microti* and *Babesia duncani.*

- ZYTO and other types of bioenergetic testing devices may be more useful than lab tests for confirming a diagnosis, since they can detect the presence of organisms based on their energetic frequencies, and can detect species of *Babesia* for which no lab tests have yet been developed. As with *Bartonella*, however, a *Babesia* diagnosis should be based first and foremost upon symptoms.

Treating *Babesia*

- Treating *Babesia* is crucial for recovery from Lyme disease. Treating other tick-borne infections matters, but perhaps not as much as *Babesia*, as it causes major symptoms and severely compromises the immune system.

- Lyme disease symptoms are worse in people who are co-infected with *Babesia*.

- For some people, taking Mepron (atovaquone) along with azithromycin is no longer sufficient for treating *Babesia* infections, since they are fast becoming resistant to these and other medications. Taking different or additional medications, such as Septra or Malarone, may be better for some.

- According to Richard Horowitz, MD, when Mepron and Zithromax (azithromycin) prove insufficient for treating *Babesia*, rotating other combinations of antibiotics and antimalarial medications may be more effective (for example, adding Septra to Mepron and Zithromax;

or rotating between Mepron to Malarone at increased dosing, and combining these with either Artemisia or Cryptolepis). While Dr. Horowitz doesn't often use Cleocin and quinine due to their more serious side effects, sometimes combining Cleocin with a macrolide such as Zithromax can be effective. Intravenous clindamycin may also be beneficial for patients who have failed oral treatment regimens. Artemether and Coartem are other *Babesia* treatment options that may work when other treatments fail.

- According to Dr. Horowitz, it is becoming necessary to use increasingly higher doses of anti-*Babesia* medications to effectively combat *Babesia* infections.

- As with other tick-borne pathogens, a number of *Babesia* organisms may remain in the body after several years of treatment. Treatment regimens should be undertaken until all symptoms disappear.

- Herbal remedies are also useful for treating *Babesia*. Combining them with anti-malarial medications may be the most beneficial treatment strategy. Cryptolepis and Artemisia are two of the most common herbal remedies used to treat this infection.

- For complete, updated guidelines on how to treat Babesia, check out Dr. Horowitz's 2011 ILADS presentation which can be obtained from the ILADS website: www.ilads.org.

Lyme Disease Treatment Considerations

- Herxheimer (detoxification) reactions increase inflammation. This inflammation can further upset homeostasis (equilibrium) in the body and can be harmful if not adequately treated. Overly aggressive antibiotic regimens can cause significant setbacks in healing; however, gentle antibiotic regimens promote antibiotic resistance, so it's important to find a happy medium between the two approaches. The best way to manage a severe Herxheimer reaction is by temporarily interrupting treatment.

- Treatment failures can be due to many things, including taking or giving the wrong antibiotic doses, administering treatment for an inappropriate period of time, or administering an incomplete antibiotic/herbal regimen.

- If a patient has a poor response to treatment, it's important for the doctor to consider whether: 1) the diagnosis is correct; 2) there may be other co-infections in the person's body that aren't being treated; 3) other concurrent illnesses are causing symptoms; 4) the antibiotic regimen is appropriate for the diagnosis and stage of disease (some drug combinations may need to be changed); 5) the medication doses are high enough; 6) the patient requires IV therapy instead of oral medication; and 7) the treatments need to be done for a longer period of time.

- Challenges to effective Lyme disease treatment include: 1) compromised immune function; 2) a genetic inability to detoxify; 3) inflammation; 4) a lack of enzymatic activity in the gut; 5) nutritional deficiencies; 6) emotional trauma; 7) a lack of financial resources; and 8) the fact that most people have many infections, including viruses, mycoplasmas, protozoa, parasites, biofilms, chlamydias, and others.

- Intravenous immunoglobulin (IVIG) treatments may be beneficial for people with Lyme disease who still have severe neuropathic symptoms after their infections have been controlled. Such symptoms include: pain, autonomic nervous system dysfunction (e.g., dysautonomias, ortheostasis, GI dysfunction, and air hunger). IVIG can reverse some of these symptoms, aid in the re-myelineation of nerves, and lower inflammation.

- Heavy metals, mitochondrial dysfunction, and adrenal fatigue all suppress the immune system and render treatments for Lyme infections less effective or ineffective.

- Intravenous glutathione lowers inflammatory cytokines (and may therefore be a helpful adjunct to treatment).

- During treatment, it's important to reduce as many stressors as possible, particularly insomnia and pain. Doing whatever you need to do to get the immune system back in charge is important for recovery.

- If you can effectively treat the top three most immune-disruptive infections, the body will often heal. It is usually not necessary to eliminate all secondary infections. For most people, immune system function should normalize after treating the most important three or four infections.

Symptoms and Treatments for Other Lyme Disease Co-Infections and Opportunistic Infections

Common Lyme disease co-infections and opportunistic infections that Lyme-literate doctors test for, in addition to *Babesia* (especially the *duncani* and *microti* species, although many others exist) and *Bartonella* (especially *henslae* and *quintana*, although other species exist), include: *Mycoplasma* (especially *fermentans* and *pneumonia*), tularemia, Rocky Mountain spotted fever, *Brucella*, q-fever, Powassen virus, *Chlamydia*, herpes viruses, *Helicobacter pylori* (and other parasites), and coxsackie virus.

Mycoplasma

- *Mycoplasma* causes chronic fatigue syndrome, arthralgia, insomnia, fever, fatigue, encephalitis, and meningitis.
- Treatments include macrolide, quinolone, or tetracycline-type antibiotics. Sulfa-type drugs may also be useful.
- Chlamydia
- Lyme disease patients who are very ill almost always have *Chlamydia pneumonia* infections.
- Treatments include: doxycycline, azithromycin, and rifampin.

Human Monocytic Ehrlichiosis

- Symptoms include: fever, vomiting, neurological symptoms, and sometimes cough and rashes. People with this infection also often have fibromyalgia-like symptoms, soft tissue pain, recurrent tendonitis, and severe headaches.
- Leukopenia (low white blood cell counts) and thrombocytopenia (low platelet counts) may also be present.
- Treatments include a combination of doxycycline and rifampin. Quinolone-type antibiotics have some efficacy in vitro and may work when the latter fail.

Anaplasmosis

- Symptoms of anaplasmosis include anorexia, arthralgia (joint pain), nausea, cough, leukopenia, atypical pneumonia, and thrombocytopenia.
- Treatment includes tetracyclines, rifampin and levofloxacin.

Treating Lyme Disease Infections with Herbal Remedies

- Herbal remedies can be used as a standalone treatment for tick-borne infections, or in conjunction with antibiotics.

- Combination herbal formulas and protocols can be especially effective for people with antibiotic-resistant infections.

- In addition to having antibacterial, antiparasitic, antifungal, and antiviral properties, herbs are multifaceted in their ability to help the body to heal. They aid in detoxification, are high in nutrients and antioxidants, and support organ function. Herbal remedies are useful not only for eliminating microbes, but also for supporting immune function and other systems of the body.

- According to Jeffrey Wulfman, MD, in a 2011 ILADS meeting presentation, herbal remedies are most effective/useful when: 1) a patient relapses on antibiotic treatments; 2) the patient has a weak/depleted vitality or constitution; and 3) the illness is (to quote Wulfman), "slow and smoldering." According to Dr. Wulfman, antibiotics tend to be a better choice for: 1) people who have rapidly escalating symptoms; 2) those who have heavy neurological involvement in their overall symptom picture; 3) people who are in the early stages of illness (acute Lyme); 4) children and the elderly; 5) people with fewer cofactors (e.g., infections); and 6) those with a good pre-existing vitality.

- People have various responses to pharmaceutical antibiotics. In some cases, they can be life-saving, but not in others. Where they are harmful or only minimally helpful, herbal remedies may be a better choice of treatment.

- Sue McCamish, CTN, has created a variety of herbal remedies that are being used by many Lyme-literate healthcare practitioners for tick-borne and other infections. Her remedies also address immune function, detoxification, enzymatic activity and biofilms, among other things. For more information on these remedies, visit www. saliva-testing.org.

- One advantage to using herbs for treating infections, instead of antibiotics, is that they don't increase the risk of developing fungal infections that are associated with long-term antibiotic use. Also, unlike antibiotics, they don't deplete the body's healthy gastrointestinal and immune-protective bacteria.

Lyme Disease and Pregnancy

- According to Charles Ray Jones, MD, if a pregnant woman with Lyme disease takes two antibiotics while pregnant, the chances that she will transmit Lyme to her baby are less than one percent. If she takes only one antibiotic, that percentage rises to 25 percent.
- A mother with Lyme should breast-feed her baby only if she is on antibiotics, since spirochetes live in breast milk.
- A 1995 study revealed that if a pregnant woman with Lyme disease doesn't take antibiotics during her pregnancy, there is a 67 percent chance that she will transmit Lyme disease to her baby.
- It is uncertain whether a father can pass Lyme disease on to his child, but it has been proven that he can pass it to his wife, who can then pass it on to their child.
- Permanent damage to the fetus can occur if a pregnant woman with Lyme disease isn't treated with antibiotics during her pregnancy.
- Lyme can't be transmitted via cow's milk or other animal's milk because spirochetes can't live for long when exposed to air, and thus die in the milking process.

Supportive Treatments

Exercise

- Exercise is critical for recovery.
- Some Lyme-literate doctors advocate not doing aerobic exercise until the tick-borne infections have been adequately controlled. Weight and resistance training and Pilates are often better types of exercise for those with chronic Lyme disease.
- Exercise should not be done daily, as this will stress the adrenal glands too much. Ideally, it should be performed every other day.

Dietary Recommendations

Lyme-literate doctors differ somewhat in their ideas about what constitutes an ideal diet for people with Lyme disease. Many say that a low-glycemic diet is important, as is avoiding food allergies. Common food allergens include: corn, soy, gluten, dairy, grains, sugar, eggs, and peanuts.

Information on IDSA versus ILADS Treatment Guidelines

According to the Infectious Diseases Society of America (IDSA), chronic Lyme disease most likely does not exist. The organization contends that Lyme disease symptoms are most likely the aches and pains of daily living. They also contend that there is little evidence for persistent infection, and that treatments for chronic Lyme disease are therefore ineffective. The IDSA acknowledges the existence of acute Lyme disease, however, and believes that 10–20 days of antibiotic treatment is sufficient for treating it. According to their guidelines, most people with Lyme disease have an erythema migrans rash when they are bitten by a tick, along with symptoms of heart block, meningitis, and arthritis.

Unfortunately, the IDSA recommendations are based on flawed guidelines that were established by the National Institutes of Health (NIH). IDSA has dismissed extensive studies and clinical evidence from scientists and clinicians that proves the existence of chronic Lyme disease and the effectiveness of prolonged antibiotic treatment regimens. Thus, IDSA guidelines are based upon a failure to use rigorous testing methodologies, poor scientific studies, and unmanaged conflicts of interest among those responsible for making the guidelines.

On the other hand, the International Lyme and Associated Diseases Society (ILADS) guidelines are based upon the work of over seventeen doctors, and are supported by over 800 references that take into account: 1) patient exposure to Lyme; 2) evidence of persistent infection; 3) mechanisms of persistent infection; 4) clinical presentation of symptoms; 5) diagnostic evaluation; 6) lab findings; 7) treatment options; 8) prevention, and 9) research.

Lyme disease is associated with the presence of many infections. It is difficult to diagnose, and symptoms can be severe. It can also be difficult and costly to treat, and can persist for years in the body.

Appendix II

Babesia and *Bartonella* Symptoms and Indicators
By James Schaller, MD

(For more information on these infections, see Dr. Schaller's website: www.personal-consult.com, where his many books on these and other infections and conditions can be either purchased or downloaded for free).

Babesia Symptoms and Indicators

All of the following can indicate the presence of a *Babesia* infection:

1. Reacting to any derivative of Artemisia (sweet wormwood).

2. Reacting to malaria drugs. It requires profound wisdom for a clinician to be able to distinguish between a side effect of a medication and a (Herxheimer) reaction caused by an effective *Babesia* treatment. For example, insomnia caused by the synthetic drug Larium is meaningless, since Larium causes this side effect in uninfected patients. But fatigue and a severe headache that result from taking a teaspoon of Mepron on day one of treatment are symptoms that indicate a protozoan-like *Babesia*, malarial, or other similar type of infection.

3. Headaches with no clear cause.

4. Headaches that are hard to control.

5. Weight gain in clear excess of (or disproportionate to) a person's diet and exercise.

6. Weight loss with reasonable eating and average exercise.

7. Fatigue in excess of that experienced by most people within the same age range.

8. Fatigue that produces a need for sleep in excess of 8.5 hours daily.

9. Fatigue with ongoing insomnia (consider the possibility that both *Bartonella* and *Babesia* are present whenever this is the case).

10. Absolute Eosinophils in the low or high range on lab tests (this test should not be used to establish a definitive diagnosis, but is a useful tool for helping to confirm one).

11. A percentage of Eosinophils in the low or high normal range on lab tests.

12. Very high Eosinophils (this is rare with *Babesia*, as research suggests other possible causes).

13. Mood changes when taking any herb or drug (except Larium) that kills protozoa-like *Babesia*.

14. Shortness of breath when the person has no obvious asthma, pneumonia, COPD, or another common cause of this symptom.

15. Swelling in the limbs and other parts of the body.

16. Night sweats.

17. Excessive perspiration during normal daily activity.

18. Hot flashes in a normal temperature room.

19. Poor appetite.

20. Intermittent fever.

21. Chills.

22. High fever.

23. A high fever which lasts longer than three days.

24. Slowed thinking.

25. Listlessness.

26. A normal or low VEGF lab result when *Bartonella* is also present.

27. A TNF-a lab test result in excess of 1.0 when *Bartonella* is also present.

28. A CD57 or CD57/8 level that drops right after the start of a *Babesia* treatment, or which falls steadily with ongoing treatment.

29. Pets, farm animals, or local relatives with any tick-borne virus, bacteria, or protozoa.

30. In men or boys, excess breast tissue.

31. Decreased appetite.

32. Severe chest wall pains.

33. Random stabbing pains.

34. Any enhanced sensitivity to light, touch, smells, or sound.

35. Family, friends, or others report that you, the sick person, look tired or seem foggy.

36. You have received blood from another person.

37. Muscle aches or joint aches/pain, which worsen after using protozoa-killing medications such as proquanil, Alinia, atovaquone, clindamycin, or one of the many new, emerging progressive natural medicine or synthetic malaria drug treatments.

38. Nausea or vomiting.

39. Hemolytic anemia with positive lab tests revealing blood products in the urine (this is not a routine finding, however).

40. Dark urine (although this is rarer than some articles have indicated).

41. An enlarged liver.

42. An enlarged spleen.

43. A yellow hue on the eyes, hands, and skin (jaundice) with no other clear cause.

44. Sexual contact is a debated form of transmission for some tick- and flea-borne infections. I (Dr. Schaller) take no position on the issue. The presence of pathogens in a body fluid does not mean that that particular fluid is a vector for spreading the infection. If you (the patient) and your healer feel that body fluids are vectors for transmission, it's important to consider whether you have intimately shared body fluids with an infected person.

45. The patient's mother is suspected of having, or has been diagnosed with *Babesia*, *Ehrlichia*, Rocky Mountain spotted fever, Anaplasma, Lyme, or

Bartonella, based on newer direct and indirect testing methods, or clinical signs and symptoms.

46. A sibling, father, spouse, or child with any tick-borne infection who shared a residence or vacation in a wooded area.

47. Exposure to outdoor environments containing brush, wild grasses, wild streams, golf courses, or woods, and which are within the vicinity of any location lived or visited since eighteen months of age.

48. Outdoor exposure to locations such as brush, wild grasses, wild streams, or woods, without having used DEET or very high off-gassing essential oils on exposed skin areas.

49. Enlarged lymph nodes (this is also seen in people with *Borrelia* and *Bartonella*, and whenever a person has other infections, high inflammation, tumors, and other diseases).

50. Increased IL-6 levels following *Babesia* treatment.

51. Cognitive difficulties, such as trouble keeping up with past routine life demands; lateness due to trouble with motivation and organization, and trouble with concentration (any of these may indicate *Babesia*).

52. Memory problems, although in and of itself, this symptom does not specifically indicate a single infection or disease process. For example, exposure to indoor mold's biological chemicals can decrease memory within an hour, depending upon the species of mold that is present.

53. Profound psychiatric illness (this can be caused by things other than *Babesia*, as well).

54. Daytime sleep urgency, despite adequate nighttime sleep.

55. Waves of generalized itching (this sign of infection and inflammation isn't just limited to *Babesia*).

56. A fever which exceeds 100.5 degrees, and which sometimes occurs after a tick bite.

57. Insomnia after taking a malaria-killing herb or drug.

58. Anxiety and/or depression after taking a malaria-killing herb or drug.

59. Rage or temporary personality regression immediately after using a malaria-killing herb or medication.

60. Excess fat in the lower belly area that is in excess of (or disproportionate to) lifestyle and activity.

61. Lumps or other types of tissue collection on the body that have no clear cause (other tick- and flea-borne infections can also cause these growths).

62. One or more medical problems with unclear cause(s), changing or contradictory diagnoses, or which are eventually labeled "idiopathic."

63. Psychiatric label(s) (diagnoses) given by other practitioners as an excuse for all of your troubles or a child's or relative's troubles, when abnormal laboratory results indicate that other medical problems are the cause of psychiatric symptoms.

64. Infection with two or more tick- or flea-borne viruses, bacteria, or protozoa. The presence of other infections, such as tick-borne viruses or bacteria, should cause one to suspect that *Babesia* may also be present.

65. Your health care practitioner understands how to use indirect testing methods and believes that your lab test patterns suggest the presence of a *Babesia* infection.

66. Since direct tests for *Babesia* (by any lab) miss many human species of the organism, are of variable reliability, and the common co-presence of *Bartonella* suppresses some antibody tests for *Babesia*, a positive or "indeterminate" result on a lab test for *Babesia* is more likely to be a positive.

67. You have neighbors living near you who have been diagnosed with tick- or flea-borne infections.

68. Your pet(s) or family animals of any type (e.g., horses) have been exposed to outdoor areas such as brush, wild grasses, wild streams, or woods, but were not given regularly scheduled anti-tick and anti-flea treatments.

69. Clear exposure as an adult to ticks in your current or past homes.

70. Clear exposure to ticks during vacations or other travels.

Bartonella Symptoms and Indicators

1. Insomnia (unless there is also profound fatigue, in which case this symptom might not apply to people with *Bartonella*).

2. Current anxiety or depression that was not present at age ten or twenty (if you are an adult).

3. Knee-jerk emotional responses which are worse than they were in past decades and which continue to worsen.

4. Unusual discomfort on the soles of your feet.

5. A temperature under 98.3 in a person who is sick. A temperature under 99.0 if Lyme disease or *Babesia* are also present.

6. Puffy tissue on the insoles or any part of the ankles.

7. Depression.

8. Depression that is not fully controlled, or which does not improve with treatment.

9. Gingivitis or bleeding during flossing.

10. Anxiety that is poorly controlled, despite average dosing of anti-anxiety treatments.

11. Depression that is poorly controlled, despite reasonable trials of medication.

12. Sleep medicines that work poorly at routine doses.

13. Rage that gets worse over time.

14. Irritability that gets worse over time.

15. Low IL-6 levels.

16. Low IL-1B levels.

17. TNF-a scores that are within the lower 10 percent of the normal range on lab tests.

18. Any skin markings or growths that are greater (more obvious) than most people's.

19. Blood vessels that are more obvious or bigger in size than most people's.

20. Greater impatience when compared to ten years ago (in a child, this may manifest as irritability).

21. Cursing or hostile speech that gets worse over time.

22. One or more medical problem with unclear cause(s) and which is considered to be "idiopathic."

23. Red papules of any size.

24. Skin tags, including ones that have been removed by a dermatologist or shaved off.

25. Unusually-sized blood vessels or an unusual amount of blood vessels of any kind, including those that are located inside of the organs, such as the bladder or intestinal walls.

26. Any skin finding, such as a mole, the numbers of which exceed that of most humans (e.g., 50 moles on the back).

27. Skin findings that indicate an increase in blood vessel size.

28. Increased tissue formation that manifests as skin tags, a hard plaque on the skin, or raised brown, black or red papules.

29. Blood vessels that are too large or too numerous for the location of the blood vessels; for example, when the thigh or calf has very thick surface blood vessels, or the legs, upper arms, or shoulders have explosions of many fine blood vessels.

30. Increased addictions that are more resistant to recovery than the average.

31. Increased impulsivity when compared to past years.

32. Burning skin sensations (this may have many causes, however).

33. Itching that has no clear cause and which is hard to control and remove.

34. Skin erosion that has no clear cause (such as a fire or chemical burn).

35. Minor cuts or scratches that heal slowly.

36. Slow healing from surgery.

37. Exposure to cats and dogs in excess of very incidental, rare contact.

38. The patient's mother is suspected to have *Bartonella* based on newer direct and indirect types of testing.

39. A sibling, father, or spouse with any tick- or flea-borne infection who shared a residence or vacation home that was near to brush.

40. Exposure to outdoor environments that contain brush, wild grasses, wild streams, golf courses, or woods, especially when DEET or very high off-gassing essential oils were not used on exposed skin areas.

41. Outdoor exposure to brush, wild grasses, wild streams, or woods without having used Permethrin on shoes, socks, and all clothing.

42. Clear exposure to lice, fleas, or ticks. (*Bartonella* is transmitted by a huge number of carriers, but for now, the percentage of insects that carry *Bartonella* is unknown. Furthermore, the capacity to detect all new species in all types of vectors or infected humans doesn't exist or isn't routinely available in both large and specialty labs).

43. Stretch marks in eccentric locations (e.g., arms, upper side under the armpit, around the armpit, or on the back).

44. Stretch marks that are red, pink, purple, or dark blue in color.

Recommended Reading, References and Resources

Chapter One: Adrenal Insufficiency and Hypothyroidism

Books

Bowthorpe, J. (2011) *Stop The Thyroid Madness.* Fredericksburg, TX: Laughing Grape Publishing, LLC.

Durrant-Peatfield, B. (2008) *Your Thyroid and How to Keep It Healthy.* London, UK: Hammersmith Press Limited.

Jefferies, W. (2004) *Safe Uses of Cortisol.* Springfield, IL: Charles C Thomas Pub, Ltd.

Lam, M and D. (2012) *Adrenal Fatigue Syndrome - Reclaim Your Energy and Vitality with Clinically Proven Natural Programs.* Loma Linda, CA: Adrenal Institute Press.

Poesnecker, G. (1993) *Chronic Fatigue Unmasked.* Richlandtown, PA: Humanitarian Publishing Company.

Wilson, J. (2001) *Adrenal Fatigue: The 21ˢᵗ Century Stress Syndrome* Smart Publications

Websites

Michael Lam, MD: www.drlam.com

Adrenal Supplements: www.supplementclinic.com

Stop The Thyroid Madness: www.stopthethyroidmadness.com

James Wilson, MD's adrenal fatigue website: www.adrenalfatigue.org.

Canary Club (for adrenal and thyroid hormone testing): www.canary-club.org.

Chapter Two: Nutrient Deficiencies and Toxic Food

Books

Cordain, L. (2011) *The Paleo Diet Cookbook* Hoboken, NJ: John Wiley and Sons, Inc.

Kane, P., et al. (2007) *The Detoxx Book: Detoxification of Biotoxins in Chronic Neurotoxic Syndromes.*

Pollan, M. (2009) *Food Rules.* New York, NY: Penguin Group.

Pollan, M. (2006) *The Omnivore's Dilemma.* New York, NY: Penguin Group.

Rubin, J. (2011) *Live Beyond Organic.* Kansas City, MO: Beyond Organic

Rubin, J. (2005) *The Maker's Diet* Lake Mary, CA: Siloam

Schwarzbein, D. (2002) *The Schwarzbein Principle II* Deerfield Beach, FL: Health Communications, Inc.

Singleton, K. (2008) *The Lyme Disease Solution.* Dallas, Texas: Brown Books Publishing Group.

Websites

Julianne's Paleo Zone Nutrition blog: www.paleozonenutrition.com

Better Health Guy website: www.betterhealthguy.com

Supplements:

CORE minerals: www.biopureus.com

Articles

Cummins, J. (2001, March) Toxicology Symposium, University of Guelph. Ontario, Canada. Retrieved on Dec. 10, 2011 from: http://www.psrast.org/jcfateofgen.htm

David, D., et al. (2004) Changes in USDA Food Composition Data for 43 Garden Crops, 1950 to 199. *Journal of the American College of Nutrition.* Vol. 23, No. 6 669-652

Food Commission, UK. (Jan.-March, 2006) United Kingdom: Meat and dairy: Where have all the minerals gone? *Food Magazine.* Retrieved on

December 1, 2011, from: www.foodcomm.org.uk.

Mercola, J. (2010, July). Genetically-Engineered Soybeans May Cause Allergies. *Mercola.com.* Retrieved on Dec. 13, 2011 from: http://articles. mercola.com/sites/articles/archive/2010/07/08/genetically-engineered-soybeans-may-cause-allergies.aspx

Mercola, J. (2011, Sept.)Why Are Toxin Proteins Genetically Engineered Into Your Food? *Mercola.com.* Retrieved on Jan. 3, 2011 from: http:// articles.mercola.com/sites/articles/archive/2011/09/26/why-are-toxin-proteins--genetically-engineered-into-your-food.aspx.

Pollan, M. (2002, March) Power Steer. *The New York Times.* Retrieved on November 20, 2011 from: *http://www.nytimes.com/2002/03/31/magazine/ power-ste.*

Rice, L. et. al, (2007) Soy Isoflavones Exert Differential Effects on Androgen Responsive Genes in LNCaP Human Prostate Cancer Cells. *Journal of Nutrition.* Retrieved Jan., 20122, from: *http://jn.nutrition.org/ content/137/4/964.full*

Open Letter from World Scientists to All Governments Concerning GMOs. (2000) Retrieved from the Institute of Science and Society website: http://www.i-sis.org.uk/list.php.

Role of the Insulin-Like Growth Factor Family in Cancer Development and Progression. (2000). *Journal of the National Cancer Institute.* Vol. 92, issue 18. Pp. 1472-1489. Retrieved on November 20, 2011 from: *http://jnci.oxfordjournals.org/content/92/18/1472.fuller. html?pagewanted=all&src=pm*

United States: Vegetables Without Vitamins (2001, March) *Life Extension Magazine.* Retrieved on March 1, 2012 from: http://www.lef.org/ magazine/mag2001/mar2001_report_vegetables.html

Chapter Three: Electromagnetic Radiation/Pollution

Books

Crofton, K. (2010) *Wireless Radiation Rescue.* Global Wellbeing Books

Ober, C., Sinatra, S. and Zucker, M. (2010) *Earthing: The Most Important Health Discovery Ever?* Laguna Beach, CA: Basic Health Publications.

Rees, Camilla. (2009) *Public Health SOS; The Shadow Side of The Wireless Revolution.* Charlestown, SC: Create Space.

Articles

Carlo, G. (2007). The Hidden Dangers of Cell Phone Radiation. *Life Extension Magazine.* Retrieved on March 7, 2012 from: http://www.lef.org/magazine/mag2007/aug2007_report_cellphone_radiation_01.htm

Cherry, Neil. (2002-2005). Epidemiological Studies of Enhanced Brain/CNS Cancer Incidence and Mortality from EMR and EMF Exposures. Lincoln University, Canterbury, NZ.

Cherry, Neil. (2002-2005). Evidence that EMF/EMR Causes Leukaemia/Lymphoma in Adults and Children. Lincoln University, Canterbury, NZ.

EMR Stop. (2010).Transcript Interview with Dr. Thomas M. Rau of the Paracelsus Clinic. Retrieved on Jan. 12, 2011 from: http://www.emrstop.org/index.php?option=com_content&view=article&id=139:transcript-interview-with-dr-thomas-m-rau-of-the-swiss-paracelsus-clinic&catid=6:K.(2010) www.emrstop.org

Fauteux, A. Electromagnetic Intolerance Elucidated. *EMFacts Consultancy.* Retrieved on Feb. 7, 2011 from: http://www.emfacts.com/2012/01/electromagnetic-intolerance-elucidated/

Mercola, J. Does Your Cell Phone Fall At The Bottom of the Heap for Safety? *Mercola.com.* Retrieved on Feb. 10, 2011 from: http://products.mercola.com/blue-tube-headset/.

Study Links Power Lines to Cancer (2005). *British Medical Journal.* Retrieved on March 4, 2011 from: http://www.powerlinefacts.com/large_study_links_power_lines_to_leukemia.htm.

Websites

The Institute of Building Biology + Ecology Neubeuern: http://www.baubiologie.de/site/english.php

Electromagnetic Health (website of Camilla Rees, MBA): www.electromagnetichealth.org

French Association for Research in Therapeutics against Cancer: www.artac.info

Stan Hartman, RadSafe, Boulder, Colorado: www.radsafe.net

To do an antennae search: www.antennasearch.com

Products

Earthing products: www.earthinginstitute.net

Electrosensor and other EMF products: www.lessemf.com/gauss.html

EMF Safety Store: www.emfsafetystore.com

Graham-Stetzer filters: www.stetzerelectric.com

Memon products: www.memonyourharmony.com

Chapter Four: Mold and Mycotoxins

Books

Schaller, J. (2006) *Mold Illness and Mold Remediation Made Simple (Discount Black & White Edition): Removing Mold Toxins from Bodies and Sick Buildings.* Tampa, FL: Hope Academic Press.

Shoemaker, R. (2011) *Surviving Mold: Life in the Era of Dangerous Buildings.* Otter Bay Books

Shoemaker, R. (2005) *Mold Warriors.* Baltimore, MD: Gateway Press, Inc.

Websites and On-Line Reports

Richard Loyd, PhD: www.royalrife.com/mold_toxins.pdf

James Schaller, MD: www.personalconsult.com

Ritchie Shoemaker, MD: www.survivingmold.com

Shoemaker, R., et al: *Policy Holders of America: Research Committee Report on Diagnosis and Treatment of Chronic Inflammatory Response Syndrome Caused by Exposure to the Interior Environment of Water-Damaged Buildings (2010):* Pokomoke, Maryland. Retrieved on May 1, 2012 from: http://www.survivingmold.com/legal-resources/publications/poa-position-statement-paper.

For Mold Testing

Environmental Health Center of Dallas: www.ehcd.com

ERMI-DNA Mold Testing: www.ermimoldtest.com

Real Time Labs: www.realtimelab.com

Products

Aroma-Pro Cold Air Diffuser: www.royalrife.com, http://www.essentials4health.biz/products/diffusers.shtml

Austin Air hepa filters: www.austinair.com

Cholestepure: http://www.pureencapsulations.com/itemdy00.asp?T1=CHP1

Nikken air filters: http://www.nikken.com/product/technology/air-wellness

NutraMedix' Banderol and other products: www.nutramedix.com

Thieves' oil: www.secretofthieves.com

Articles

Solfrizzo M, et al. (2001) In vitro and in vivo studies to assess the effectiveness of cholestyramine as a binding agent for fumonisins. *Mycopathologia,* 147-153. Retrieved on April 10, 2012 from: http://www.usmoldphysician.com/articles/comparingmoldtoxinbinders.html.

Chapter Five: Pyroluria/Heavy Metal Toxicity

Books

Cutler, A. (1999, June) *Amalgam Illness: Diagnosis and Treatment.* Andrew Hall Cutler; 1st edition.

Gordon, G. and Brown, D. (2007) *Detox with Oral Chelation: Protecting Yourself from Lead, Mercury, & Other Environmental Toxins.* Petaluma, CA: Smart Publications.

Articles

Hoffer, A. (1995) The Discovery of Kryptopyrrole and its Importance in Diagnosis of Biochemical Imbalances in Schizophrenia and in Criminal Behavior. *The Journal of Orthomolecular Medicine*, Vol. 10(1):3

Roberts, James. *Chelation Therapy.* Heartfixer: www.heartfixer.com. Retrieved on February 10, 2012 from: http://www.heartfixer.com/CHC%20-%20Treatments%20-%20Chelation%20Therapy.htm

Websites

Direct Health Care Access II Laboratory: http://kryptopyrrole.com/

Andrew Hall Cutler's website: www.noamalgam.com

James Roberts' website: www.heartfixer.com

Nutritional Healing: http://www.nutritional-healing.com.au/content/articles-content.php?heading=Pyroluria.

Chapter Six: Parasites

Books

Gittleman, Ann Louise (2001) *Guess What Came to Dinner? Parasites and Your Health.* New York, NY: Penguin Group, Inc.

Yu, Simon. (2010) *Accidental Cure: Extraordinary Medicine for Extraordinary Patients.* St. Louis, MO: Prevention and Healing, Inc.

Articles and Conference References

Oz, Mehmet. (2006) Dr. Oz Answers Your Questions. *Oprah.com.* Retrieved on April 2, 2012 from: http://www.oprah.com/health/Dr-Oz-Answers-Burning-Medical-Questions2), Mar 1997, 171-191

Watkins, W. Pollitt, E. (1997, March) "Stupidity or worms": Do intestinal worms impair mental performance? *Psychological Bulletin,* Vol 121(2), 171-191.

Yu, Simon. (2011, May) Accidental Cure: Think Parasites and Dental Problems when the Latest Medical Therapies Failed. Conference, "A Deep Look Beyond Lyme": Bellevue, Washington.

Products

ReNew Life's ParaGone: www.renewlife.com/paragone.html

Parastroy: www.naturessecret.com/products/parastroy

Humaworm: http://humaworm.com

Chapter Seven: Gastrointestinal Dysfunction

Books

Barron, J. (2008) *Lessons from The Miracle Doctors: A Step-by-Step Guide to Optimum Health and Relief from Catastrophic Illness.* Basic Health Publications

Mullin, G., Swift, K.M., and Weil, A., (2011) *The Inside Tract: Your Good Gut Guide to Great Digestive Health* Emmaus, PA: Rodale Books

Articles

Barron, J. (1999-2012) Digestive Problems and Alternative Remedies. *Baseline of Health Foundation.* Retrieved on March 24, 2012 from: http://www.jonbarron.org/natural-health/remedies-digestive-disorders

Mercola, J. (2011, Oct) Is Leaky Gut Causing You to Pack on The Pounds? *Mercola.com.* Retrieved on April 16, 2011 from: http://articles.mercola.com/sites/articles/archive/2011/10/12/is-a-leaky-gut-causing-you-to-pack-on-the-pounds.aspx

Websites

Barron, J. *Baseline of Health Foundation*: www.jonbarron.org

Cowden Support Program and NutraMedix: www.nutramedix.com

Leaky Gut Syndrome website: www.leakygut.co.uk

Researched Nutritionals: www.researchednutritionals.com

Products

Prescript-Assist Pro: www.researchednutritionals.com

For probiotics:

Klaire Labs: www.klaire.com

VSL #3: www.vsl3.com

Custom Probiotics: www.customprobiotics.com

Chapter Eight: Emotional Trauma

Books

Emoto, M. (2005) *The Hidden Messages in Water.* New York, NY: Atria Books

Lipton, B. (2005) *The Biology of Belief.* Santa Rosa, CA: Mountain of Love/Elite Books

Loyd, A. (2010) *The Healing Code: 6 Minutes to Heal the Source of Your Health, Success, or Relationship Issue.* New York, NY: Grand Central Life & Style, Hatchette Book Group.

Myhill, S. (2010) *Diagnosing and Treating Chronic Fatigue Syndrome.* Knighton, Powys, UK: Sarah Myhill Limited.

Sahelian, R. (2000) *Mind Boosters: A Guide to Natural Supplements That Enhance Your Mind, Memory, and Mood* New York, NY: St. Martin's Griffin.

Siegel, B. (1986) *Love, Medicine and Miracles.* New York, NY: Harper and Row Publishers, Inc.

Townsend, J. and Cloud, H. (1992) *Boundaries: When to Say Yes, When to Say No to Take Control of Your Life,* Grand Rapids, MI: Zondervan.

Articles

Arai, S and Mock, S. (2011, Jan.) Childhood trauma and chronic illness in adulthood: mental health and socioeconomic status as explanatory factors and buffers. *Frontiers in Developmental Psychology.* Retrieved on March 7, 2012 from: http://www.frontiersin.org/developmental_psychology/10.3389/fpsyg.2010.00246/full

Gut Health. *Point of Return.* Retrieved on March 11, 2012 from: https://pointofreturn.com/gut_health.html.

Kendall-Tackett, K. Why Trauma Makes People Sick: Inflammation, Heart Disease and Diabetes in Trauma Survivors. *Best Thinking Medicine.* Retrieved on Feb. 17, 2012 from: http://www.bestthinking.com/articles/medicine/psychiatry_and_neurology/why-trauma-makes-people-sick-inflammation-heart-disease-and-diabetes-in-trauma-survivors

Writing Group for the Women's Health Initiative Investigators. (2002) *Risks and benefits of estrogen plus progestin in healthy postmenopausal women. Principal results from the Women's Health Initiative randomized controlled trial.* JAMA, 288:321-333.

Websites

Neuroscience: www.neurorelief.comPoint of Return: www.pointofreturn.com

Chapter Nine: Other Conditions That Contribute to Disease in People with Tick-Borne Infections

Candida

Gates, D. and Schatz, L. (2011) *The Body Ecology Diet: Recovering Your Health and Rebuilding Your Immunity.* Hay House

Teich, M. (2011, Oct.) Food Allergy, Intolerance and Candida. Presentation at Oct. 2011 International Lyme and Associated Diseases Society conference. Toronto, Ontario, Canada.

The Candida Diet website: www.thecandidadiet.com/foodstoavoid.html

Opportunistic Viruses and Bacteria

For more information on how to treat tick-borne and opportunistic infections according to ILADS guidelines, physician conference DVD presentations are available for purchase at: International Lyme and Associated Diseases Society (ILADS): http://www.ilads.org/store/store_lyme_dvd2010.html.

Structural Problems

For more information on prolotherapy visit: www.prolotherapy.org, www.prolotherapy.com

For more information on Yamuna body rolling, visit: www.yamunabody-rolling.com

For more information on Pilates, visit: http://pilates.about.com/od/whatispilates/a/WhatIsPilates.htm

Foci Infections

Cutler, A. *Amalgam Illness: Diagnosis and Treatment* (1999). Andrew Hall Cutler.

Fields, Perry (2012) *The Tick Slayer: Battling Lyme Disease and Winning.* Clemson, SC: Zippy Publishing, LLC.

Huggins (1999) *Uninformed Consent: The Hidden Dangers in Dental Care.* Newburyport, MA: Hampton Roads Publications.

Huggins, H. (2010) Root Canal Dangers. *The Weston A. Price Foundation.* Retrieved on March 18, 2012 from: *http://www.westonaprice.org/dentistry/root-canal-dangers*

P. Vernon Erwin, DDS' website: www.drerwin.com

William Glaros, DDS' website: www.biologicaldentist.com

Hal Huggins' DDS' website: www.hugginsappliedhealing.com

O'Sullivan, B. What Is a Cavitat? *Road to Health, Newsletter 70.* Retrieved on March 7, 2012 from: http://road-to-health.com/dental_osteomyelitis/What_is_a_Cavitat_.html

Lyme Disease Books

Buhner, S. H. (2005) *Healing Lyme: Natural Healing and Prevention of Lyme Borreliosis and Its Coinfections.* Randolph, VT: Raven Press.

McFadzean, N. (2010) *The Lyme Diet: Nutritional Strategies for Healing from Lyme Disease.* San Diego, CA: Legacy Line Publishing.

Rosner, Bryan (2007) *The Top 10 Lyme Disease Treatments.* S. Lake Tahoe: BioMed Publishing Group

Rosner, Bryan (2005) *When Antibiotics Fail: Lyme Disease and Rife Machines, with Critical Evaluation of Leading Alternative Therapies.* S. Lake Tahoe: BioMed Publishing Group.

Schaller, J. (2006) *The Diagnosis and Treatment of Babesia.* Hope Academic Press.

Schaller, J. (2008) *Bartonella: Diagnosis and Treatment - A Major Cause of Lyme Disease Complications and Psychiatric Problems.* Hope Academic Press.

Singleton, K. (2008) *The Lyme Disease Solution.* Dallas, TX: Brown Books Publishing Group.

Strasheim, Connie (2009) *Insights Into Lyme Disease Treatment: 13 Lyme-Literate Health Care Practitioners Share Their Healing Strategies.* S. Lake Tahoe: BioMed Publishing Group.

Weintraub, P. (2009) *Cure Unknown: Inside The Lyme Epidemic.* St. Martin's Griffin.

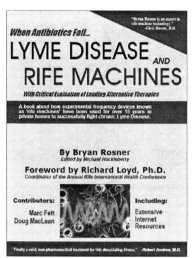

Book • $35

When Antibiotics Fail: Lyme Disease And Rife Machines, With Critical Evaluation Of Leading Alternative Therapies

By Bryan Rosner
Foreword by Richard Loyd, Ph.D.

There are enough books and websites about what Lyme disease is and which ticks carry it. But there is very little useful information for people who actually have a case of Lyme disease that is not responding to conventional antibiotic treatment. Lyme disease sufferers need to know their options, not how to identify a tick.

This book describes how experimental electromagnetic frequency devices known as rife machines have been used for over 15 years in private homes to fight Lyme disease. Also included are evaluations of more than 25 conventional and alternative Lyme disease therapies, including:

- Homeopathy
- IV and oral antibiotics
- Mercury detox.
- Hyperthermia / saunas
- Ozone and oxygen
- Samento®
- Colloidal Silver
- Bacterial die-off detox.

- Colostrum
- Magnesium supplementation
- Hyperbaric oxygen chamber (HBOC)
- ICHT Italian treatment
- Non-pharmaceutical antibiotics
- Exercise, diet and candida protocols
- Cyst-targeting antibiotics
- The Marshall Protocol®

Many Lyme disease sufferers have heard of rife machines, some have used them. But until now, there has not been a concise and organized source to explain how and why they have been used by Lyme patients. In fact, this is the first book ever published on this important topic.

The Foreword for the book is by Richard Loyd, Ph.D., coordinator of the annual Rife International Health Conference. The book takes a practical, down-to-earth approach which allows you to learn about*:

> "This book provides life-saving insights for Lyme disease patients."
>
> **- Richard Loyd, Ph.D.**

- Antibiotic treatment problems and shortcomings—why some people choose to use rife machines after other therapies fail.
- Hypothetical treatment schedules and sessions, based on the author's experience.
- The experimental machines with the longest track record: High Power Magnetic Pulser, EMEM Machine, Coil Machine, and AC Contact Machine.
- Explanation of the "herx reaction" and why it may indicate progress.
- The intriguing story that led to the use of rife machines to fight Lyme disease 20 years ago.
- Antibiotic categories and classifications, with pros and cons of each type of drug.
- Visit our website to read FREE EXCERPTS from the book!

***Disclaimer:** Your treatment decisions must be made under the care of a licensed physician. Rife machines are not FDA approved and the FDA has not reviewed or approved of these books. The author is a layperson, not a doctor, and much of the content of these books is a statement of opinion based on the author's personal experience and research.*

Paperback book, 8.5 x 11", 203 pages, $35

The Top 10 Lyme Disease Treatments: Defeat Lyme Disease With The Best Of Conventional And Alternative Medicine

By Bryan Rosner
Foreword by James Schaller, M.D.

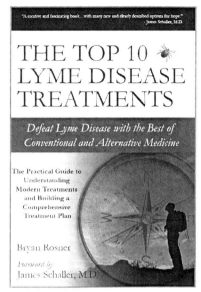

"A creative and fascinating book...with many new and clearly described options for hope."
- James Schaller, M.D.

THE TOP 10 🐞 LYME DISEASE TREATMENTS

Defeat Lyme Disease with the Best of Conventional and Alternative Medicine

The Practical Guide to
Understanding
Modern Treatments
and Building a
Comprehensive
Treatment Plan

Bryan Rosner

Foreword by
James Schaller, M.D.

Book • $35

This information-packed book identifies ten promising conventional and alternative Lyme disease treatments and gives practical guidance on integrating them into a comprehensive treatment plan that you and your physician can customize for your individual situation and needs.

The book was not written to replace Bryan Rosner's first book (*Lyme Disease and Rife Machines*, opposing page). It was written to complement that book, offering Lyme sufferers many new foundational and supportive treatment options, based on the author's extensive research and years of personal experience. Topics include*:

- Systemic enzyme therapy, which helps detoxify tissues and blood, reduce inflammation, stimulate the immune system, and kill Lyme disease bacteria.
- Lithium orotate, a powerful yet all-natural mineral (belonging to the same mineral group as sodium and potassium) capable of profound neuroprotective activity.
- Thorough and extensive coverage of a complete Lyme disease detoxification program, including discussion of both liver and skin detoxification pathways. Specific detoxification therapies such as liver cleanses, bowel cleanses, the Shoemaker Neurotoxin Elimination Protocol, sauna therapy, mineral baths, mineral supplementation, milk thistle, and many others. Ideas to reduce and control herx reactions.
- Tips and clinical research from James Schaller, M.D.
- A detailed look at one method for utilizing antibiotics during a rife machine treatment campaign.
- Wide coverage of the Marshall Protocol, including an in-depth discussion of its mechanism of action in relation to Lyme disease pathology. Also, the author's personal experience with the Marshall Protocol over 3 years.
- An explanation of and new information about the Salt / Vitamin C protocol.
- Hot-off-the-press information on mangosteen fruit (not to be confused with mango) and its many benefits, including antibacterial, anti-inflammatory, and anti-cancer properties.
- New guidelines for combining all the therapies discussed in both of Rosner's books into a complete treatment plan. Brief and articulate for consideration by you and your doctor.
- Also includes updates on rife therapy, cutting-edge supplements, political challenges, an exclusive interview with Willy Burgdorfer, Ph.D. (discoverer of Lyme), and much more!

"Bryan Rosner thinks big and this new book offers big solutions."
- James Schaller, M.D.

"Another ground-breaking Lyme Disease book."
- Jeff Mittelman, moderator of the Lyme-and-rife group

"Brilliant and thorough."
- Nenah Sylver, Ph.D.

Do not miss this top Lyme disease resource. Discover new healing tools today! Bring this book to your doctor's appointment to help with forming a treatment plan.

Paperback book, 7 x 10", 367 pages, $35

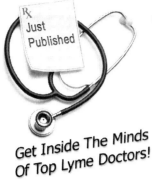

13 Lyme Doctors Share Treatment Strategies!

In this new book, not one, but thirteen Lyme-literate healthcare practitioners describe the tools they use in their practices to heal patients from chronic Lyme disease. Never before available in book format!

Get Inside The Minds Of Top Lyme Doctors!

Insights Into Lyme Disease Treatment:
13 Lyme Literate Health Care Practitioners
Share Their Healing Strategies

By Connie Strasheim
Foreword by Maureen Mcshane, M.D.

If you traveled the country for appointments with 13 Lyme-literate health care practitioners, you would discover many cutting-edge therapies used to combat chronic Lyme disease. You would also spend thousands of dollars on hotels, plane tickets, and medical appointment fees—not to mention the time it would take to embark on such a journey.

Even if you had the time and money to travel, would the physicians have enough time to answer all of your questions? Would you even know which questions to ask?

In this long-awaited book, health care journalist and Lyme patient Connie Strasheim

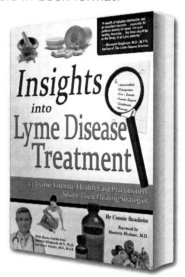

Paperback • 443 Pages • $39.95

has done all the work for you. She conducted intensive interviews with 13 of the world's most competent Lyme disease healers, asking them thoughtful, important questions, and then spent months compiling their information into 13 organized, user-friendly chapters that contain the core principles upon which they base their medical treatment of chronic Lyme disease. The practitioners' backgrounds span a variety of disciplines, including allopathic, naturopathic, complementary, chiropractic, homeopathic, and energy medicine. All aspects of treatment are covered, from anti-microbial remedies and immune system support, to hormonal restoration, detoxification, and dietary/lifestyle choices. **PHYSICIANS INTERVIEWED:**

- Steven Bock, M.D.
- Ginger Savely, DNP
- Ronald Whitmont, M.D.
- Nicola McFadzean, N.D.
- Jeffrey Morrison, M.D.
- Steven J. Harris, M.D.
- Peter J. Muran, M.D., M.B.A.

- Ingo D. E. Woitzel, M.D.
- Susan L. Marra, M.S., N.D.
- W. Lee Cowden, M.D., M.D. (H)
- Deborah Metzger, Ph.D., M.D.
- Marlene Kunold, "Heilpraktiker"
- Elizabeth Hesse-Sheehan, DC, CCN
- Visit our website to read a FREE CHAPTER!

Paperback book, 7 x 10", 443 pages, $39.95

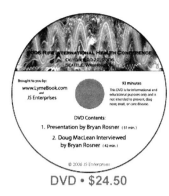

DVD • $24.50

Rife International Health Conference
Feature-Length DVD (93 Minutes)

Bryan Rosner's Presentation and Interview
with Doug MacLean

**The Official Rife Technology Seminar
Seattle, WA, USA**

If you have been unable to attend the Rife
International Health Conference, this DVD is your
opportunity to watch two very important Lyme-
related presentations from the event:

Presentation #1: Bryan Rosner's Sunday
morning talk entitled *Lyme Disease: New Paradigms in Diagnosis and Treatment -
the Myths, the Reality, and the Road Back to Health.* (51 minutes)

Presentation #2: Bryan Rosner's interview with Doug MacLean, in which Doug
talked about his experiences with Lyme disease, including the incredible journey he
undertook to invent the first modern rife machine used to fight Lyme disease.
Although Doug's journey as a Lyme disease pioneer took place 20 years ago, this
was the first time Doug has ever accepted an invitation to appear in public. This is
the only video available where you can see Doug talk about what it was like to be the
first person ever to use rife technology as a treatment for Lyme disease. Now you
can see how it all began. Own this DVD and own a piece of history! (42 minutes)

Lymebook.com has secured a special licensing agreement with JS Enterprises, the
Canadian producer of the Rife Conference videos, to bring this product to you at the
special low price of $24.50. Total DVD viewing time: 1 hour, 33 minutes. We have
DVDs in stock, shipped to you within 3 business days.

Price Comparison (should you get the DVD?)

**Cost of attending the recent
Rife Conference (2 people):**
Hotel Room, 3 Nights = $400
Registration = $340
Food = $150
Airfare = $600
Total = $1,490

**Cost of the DVD, which you can
view as many times as you want,
and show to family and friends:**
DVD = $24.50

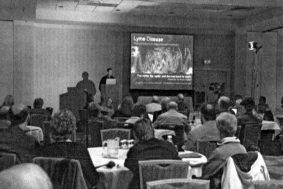

**Bryan Rosner
Presenting on
Sunday Morning
In Seattle**

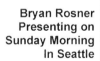

**DVD
93 Minutes
$24.50**

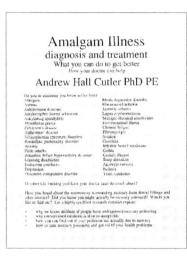

Book • $35

Amalgam Illness, Diagnosis and Treatment: What You Can Do to Get Better, How Your Doctor Can Help

By Andrew Cutler, PhD

This book was written by a chemical engineer who himself got mercury poisoning from his amalgam dental fillings. He found that there was no suitable educational material for either the patient or the physician. Knowing how much people can suffer from this condition, he wrote this book to help them get well. With a PhD in chemistry from Princeton University and extensive study in biochemistry and medicine, Andrew Cutler uses layman's terms to explain how people become mercury poisoned and what to do about it. The author's research shows that mercury poisoning can easily be cured at home with over-the-counter oral chelators – this book explains how.

In the book you will find practical guidance on how to tell if you really have chronic mercury poisoning or some other problem. Proper diagnostic procedures are provided so that sick people can decide what is wrong rather than trying random treatments. If mercury poisoning is your problem, the book tells you how to get the mercury out of your body, and how to feel good while you do that. The treatment section gives step-by-step directions to figure out exactly what mercury is doing to you and how to fix it.

> "Dr. Cutler uses his background in chemistry to explain the safest approach to treat mercury poisoning. I am a physician and am personally using his protocol on myself."
>
> **- Melissa Myers, M.D.**

Sections also explain how the scientific literature shows many people must be getting poisoned by their amalgam fillings, why such a regulatory blunder occurred, and how the debate between "mainstream" and "alternative" medicine makes it more difficult for you to get the medical help you need.

This down-to-earth book lets patients take care of themselves. It also lets doctors who are not familiar with chronic mercury intoxication treat it. The book is a practical guide to getting well. Sections from the book include:

- Why worry about mercury poisoning?
- What mercury does to you – symptoms, laboratory test irregularities, diagnostic checklist.
- How to treat mercury poisoning easily with oral chelators.
- Dealing with other metals including copper, arsenic, lead, cadmium.
- Dietary and supplement guidelines.
- Balancing hormones during the recovery process.
- How to feel good while you are chelating the metals out.
- How heavy metals cause infections to thrive in the body.
- Politics and mercury.

This is the world's most authoritative, accurate book on mercury poisoning.

Paperback book, 8.5 x 11", 226 pages, $35

Hair Test Interpretation: Finding Hidden Toxicities

By Andrew Cutler, PhD

Hair tests are worth doing because a surprising number of people diagnosed with incurable chronic health conditions actually turn out to have a heavy metal problem; quite often, mercury poisoning. Heavy metal problems can be corrected. Hair testing allows the underlying problem to be identified – and the chronic health condition often disappears with proper detoxification.

Hair Test Interpretation: Finding Hidden Toxicities is a practical book that explains how to interpret **Doctor's Data, Inc.** and **Great Plains Laboratory** hair tests. A step-by-step discussion is provided, with figures to illustrate the process and make it easy. The book gives examples using actual hair test results from real people.

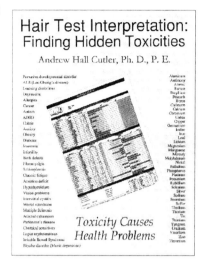

Hair Test Interpretation: Finding Hidden Toxicities

Andrew Hall Cutler, Ph. D., P. E.

Toxicity Causes Health Problems

Book • $35

One of the problems with hair testing is that both conventional and alternative health care providers do not know how to interpret these tests. Interpretation is not as simple as looking at the results and assuming that any mineral out of the reference range is a problem mineral.

Interpretation is complicated because heavy metal toxicity, especially mercury poisoning, interferes with mineral transport throughout the body. Ironically, if someone is mercury poisoned, hair test mercury is often low and other minerals may be elevated or take on unusual values. For example, mercury often causes retention of arsenic, antimony, tin, titanium, zirconium, and aluminum. An inexperienced health care provider may wrongfully assume that one of these other minerals is the culprit, when in reality mercury is the true toxicity.

"This new book of Andrew's is the definitive guide in the confusing world of heavy metal poisoning diagnosis and treatment. I'm a practicing physician, 20 years now, specializing in detoxification programs for treatment of resistant conditions. It was fairly difficult to diagnose these heavy metal conditions before I met Andrew Cutler and developed a close relationship with him while reading his books. In this book I found his usual painful attention to detail gave a solid framework for understanding the complexity of mercury toxicity as well as the less common exposures. You really couldn't ask for a better reference book on a subject most researchers and physicians are still fumbling in the dark about."
- Dr. Rick Marschall

So, as you can see, getting a hair test is only the first step. The second step is figuring out what the hair test means. Andrew Cutler, PhD, is a registered professional chemical engineer with years of experience in biochemical and healthcare research. This clear and concise book makes hair test interpretation easy, so that you know which toxicities are causing your health problems.

Paperback book, 8.5 x 11", 298 pages, $35

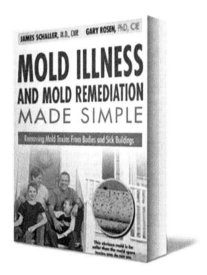

Book • $32.95

Mold Illness and Mold Remediation Made Simple: Removing Mold Toxins from Bodies and Sick Buildings

By James Schaller, M.D. and Gary Rosen, Ph.D.

Indoor mold toxins are much more dangerous and prevalent than most people realize. Visible mold in and around your house is far less dangerous than the mold you cannot see. Indoor mold toxicity, in addition to causing its own unique set of health problems and symptoms, also greatly contributes to the severity of most chronic illnesses.

In this book, a top physician and experienced contractor team up to help you quickly recover from indoor mold exposure. This book is easy to read with many color photographs and illustrations.

Dr. Schaller is a practicing physician in Florida who has written more than 15 books. He is one of the few physicians in the United States successfully treating mold toxin illness in children and adults.

Dr. Rosen is a biochemist with training under a Nobel Prize winning researcher at UCLA. He has written several books and is an expert in the mold remediation of homes. Dr. Rosen and his family are sensitive to mold toxins so he writes not only from professional experience, but also from personal experience.

Together, the two authors have certification in mold testing, mold remediation, and indoor environmental health. This book is one of the most complete on the subject, and includes discussion of the following topics:

- Potential mold problems encountered in new homes, schools, and jobs.
- Diagnosing mold illness.
- Mold as it relates to dryness and humidity.
- Mold toxins and cancer treatment.
- Mold toxins and relationships.
- Crawlspaces, basements, attics, home cleaning techniques, and vacuums.
- Training your eyes to discern indoor mold.
- Leptin and obesity.
- Appropriate/inappropriate air filters and cleaners.
- How to handle old, musty products, materials and books, and how to safely sterilize them.
- A description of various types of molds, images of them, and their relative toxicity.
- Blood testing and how to use it to find hidden health problems.
- The book is written in a friendly, casual tone that allows easy comprehension and information retention.

> "A concise, practical guide on dealing with mold toxins and their effects."
>
> **- Bryan Rosner**

Many people are affected by mold toxins. Are you? If you can find a smarter or clearer book on this subject, buy it!

Paperback book, 8.5 x 11", 140 pages, $32.95
Also available on our website as an eBook!

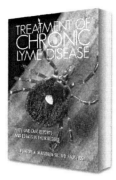

Book • $24.95

Treatment of Chronic Lyme Disease: 51 Case Reports and Essays In Their Regard

By Burton Waisbren Sr., MD, FACP, FIDSA

DON'T MISS THIS BOOK! A MUST-HAVE RESOURCE. What sets this Lyme disease book apart are the credentials of its author: he is not only a Fellow of the Infectious Diseases Society of America (IDSA), he is also one of its Founders! With 57+ years experience in medicine, Dr. Waisbren passionately argues for the validity of chronic Lyme disease and presents useful information about 51 cases of the disease which he has personally treated. His position is in stark contrast to that of the IDSA, which is a very powerful organization. **Quite possibly the most important book ever published on Lyme disease, as a result of the author's experience and credentials.**

Paperback book, 6x9", 169 pages, $24.95

Bartonella:
Diagnosis and Treatment

By James Schaller, M.D.

2 Book Set • $99.95

As an addition to his growing collection of informative books, Dr. James Schaller penned this excellent 2-part volume on Bartonella, a Lyme disease co-infection. The set is an ideal complementary resource to his Babesia textbook (next page).

Bartonella infections occur throughout the entire world, in cities, suburbs, and rural locations. It is found in fleas, dust mites, ticks, lice, flies, cat and dog saliva, and insect feces.

This 2-book set provides advanced treatment strategies as well as detailed diagnostic criteria, with dozens of full-color illustrations and photographs.

Both books in this 2-part set are included with your order.

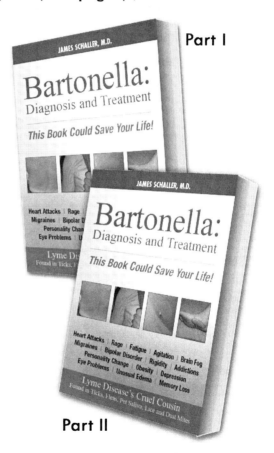

Part I

Part II

2 paperback books included, 7 x 10", 500 pages, $99.95

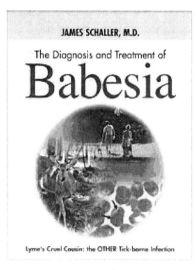

JAMES SCHALLER, M.D.

The Diagnosis and Treatment of

Babesia

Lyme's Cruel Cousin: the OTHER Tick-borne Infection

Book • $55

The Diagnosis and Treatment of Babesia: Lyme's Cruel Cousin – The Other Tick-Borne Infection

By James Schaller, M.D.

Do you or a loved one experience excess fatigue? Have you ever had unusually high fevers, chills, or sweats? You may have Babesia, a very common tick-borne infection. Babesia is often found with Lyme disease and, like all tick-borne infections, is rarely diagnosed and reported accurately.

The deer tick which carries Lyme disease and Babesia may be as small as a poppy seed and injects a painkiller, an antihistamine, and an anticoagulant to avoid detection. As a result, many people have Babesia and do not know it. Numerous forms of Babesia are carried by ticks. This book introduces patients and health care workers to the various species that infect humans and are not routinely tested for by sincere physicians.

Dr. Schaller, who practices medicine in Florida, first became interested in Babesia after one of his own children was infected with it. None of the elite pediatricians or child specialists could help. No one tested for Babesia or considered it a possible diagnosis. His child suffered from just two of these typical Babesia symptoms:

- Significant Fatigue
- Coughing
- Dizziness
- Trouble Thinking
- Fevers
- Memory Loss

- Chills
- Air Hunger
- Headache
- Sweats
- Unresponsiveness to Lyme Treatment

With 374 pages, this book is the most current and comprehensive book on Babesia in the English language. It reviews thousands of articles and presents the results of interviews with world experts on the subject. It offers you top information and broad treatment options, presented in a clear and simple manner. All treatments are explained thoroughly, including their possible side effects, drug interactions, various dosing strategies, pros/cons, and physician experiences.

"Once again Dr. Schaller has provided us with a much-needed and practical resource. This book gave me exactly what I was looking for."

- Thomas W., Patient

Finally, the book also addresses many other aspects of practical medical care often overlooked in this infection, such as treatment options for managing fatigue. Plainly stated, this book is a must-have for patients and health care providers who deal with Lyme disease and its co-infections. Dr. Schaller's many years in clinical practice give the book a practical angle that many other similar books lack. Don't miss this user-friendly resource!

Paperback book, 7 x 10", 374 pages, $55

Also available on our website as an eBook!

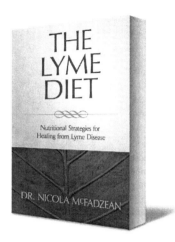

Book • $24.95

The Lyme Diet: Nutritional Strategies for Healing from Lyme Disease

By Nicola McFadzean, N.D.

We know about antibiotics and herbs. But what is the right diet for Lyme sufferers? Now you can read about the experience of Dr. Nicola McFadzean, N.D., in treating Lyme patients using proper diet.

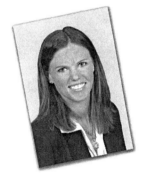

Nicola McFadzean, N.D.

The author is a Naturopathic Doctor and graduate of Bastyr University in Seattle, Washington. She is currently in private practice at her clinic, RestorMedicine, located in San Diego, California.

This book covers numerous topics (not just diet-related):

- Reducing and controlling inflammation
- Maximizing immune function via dietary choices
- Restoring the gut & regaining healthy digestion
- Detoxification with food
- Hormone imbalances
- Biofilms
- Kefir vs. yogurt vs. probiotics
- Candida, liver support, and much more!

Paperback book, 6x9", 214 Pages, $24.95
Also available as an eBook on our website!

The Stealth Killer: Is Oral Spirochetosis the Missing Link in the Dental & Heart Disease Labyrinth? *By William D. Nordquist, BS, DMD, MS*

Can oral spirochete infections cause heart attacks? In today's cosmopolitan urban population, more than 51 percent of those with root canal–treated teeth probably have infection at the apex of their root. Dr. Nordquist, an oral surgeon practicing in Southern California, believes that any source of bacteria with resulting chronic infection (including periodontal disease) in the mouth may potentially lead to heart disease and other systemic diseases. With more than 40 illustrations and x-ray reproductions, this book takes you behind the scenes in Dr. Nordquist's research laboratory, and provides many tips on dealing with Lyme-related dental problems. A breakthrough book in dentistry & infectious disease!

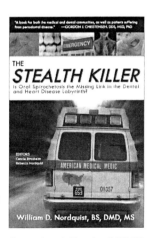

Paperback Book • $25.95

Paperback book, 6x9", 161 pages, $25.95

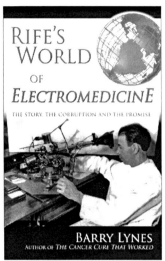

Rife's World of Electromedicine: The Story, the Corruption and the Promise

By Barry Lynes

The cause of cancer was discovered in the early 1930's. It was a virus-sized, mini-bacteria or "particle" that induced cells to become malignant and grow into tumors. The cancer microbe or particle was given the name BX by the brilliant scientist who discovered it: Royal Raymond Rife.

Laboratory verification of the cause of cancer was done hundreds of times with mice in order to be absolutely certain. Five of America's most prominent physicians helped oversee clinical trials managed by a major university's medical school.

Sixteen cancer patients were brought by ambulance twice a week to the clinical trial location in La Jolla, California. There they were treated with a revolutionary electromedicine that painlessly, non-invasively destroyed only the cancer-causing microbe or particle named BX. After just three months of this therapy, all patients were diagnosed as clinically cured. Later, the therapy was suppressed and remains so today.

In 1987, Barry Lynes wrote the classic book on Rife history (*The Cancer Cure That Worked*, see catalog page 14). *Rife's World* is the sequel.

Book • $17.95

Paperback book, 5.5 x 8.5", 90 pages, $17.95

Physicians' Desk Reference (PDR) Books (opposing page)

Most people have heard of *Physicians' Desk Reference* (PDR) books because, for over 60 years, physicians and researchers have turned to PDR for the latest word on prescription drugs.

THOMSON™

You may not know that Thomson Healthcare, publisher of PDR, offers PDR reference books not only for drugs, but also for herbal and nutritional supplements. No available books come even close to the amount of information provided in these PDRs—*PDR for Herbal Medicines* weighs 5 lbs and has over 1300 pages, and *PDR for Nutritional Supplements* weighs over 3 lbs and has more than 800 pages.

> "I relied heavily on the PDRs during the research phase of writing my books. Without them, my projects would have greatly suffered."
> **- Bryan Rosner**

We carry all three PDRs. Although PDR books are typically used by physicians, we feel that these resources are also essential for people interested in or recovering from chronic disease. For the supplements, herbs, and drugs included in the books, you will find the following information: Pharmacology, description and method of action, available trade names and brands, indications and usage, research summaries, dosage options, history of use, pharmacokinetics, and much more! Worth the money for years of faithful use.

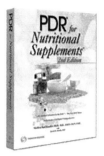

PDR for Nutritional Supplements *2ⁿᵈ Edition!*

This PDR focuses on the following types of supplements:

- Vitamins
- Minerals
- Amino acids
- Hormones
- Lipids
- Glyconutrients
- Probiotics
- Proteins
- Many more!

Book • $69.50

"In a part of the health field not known for its devotion to rigorous science, [this book] brings to the practitioner and the curious patient a wealth of hard facts."

- Roger Guillemin, M.D., Ph.D., Nobel Laureate in Physiology and Medicine

The book also suggests supplements that can help reduce prescription drug side effects, has full-color photographs of various popular commercial formulations (and contact information for the associated suppliers), and so much more! Become educated instead of guessing which supplements to take.

Hardcover book, 11 x 9.3", 800 pages, $69.50

PDR for Herbal Medicines *4ᵗʰ Edition!*

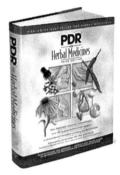

PDR for Herbal Medicines is very well organized and presents information on hundreds of common and uncommon herbs and herbal preparations. Indications and usage are examined with regard to homeopathy, Indian and Chinese medicine, and unproven (yet popular) applications.

In an area of healthcare so unstudied and vulnerable to hearsay and hype, this scientifically referenced book allows you to find out the real story behind the herbs lining the walls of your local health food store.

Use this reference before spending money on herbal products!

Book • $69.50

Hardcover book, 11 x 9.3", 1300 pages, $69.50

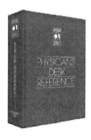

PDR for Prescription Drugs *Current Year's Edition!*

With more than 3,000 pages, this is the most comprehensive and respected book in the world on over 4,000 drugs. Drugs are indexed by both brand and generic name (in the same convenient index) and also by manufacturer and product category. This PDR provides usage information and warnings, drug interactions, plus a detailed, full-color directory with descriptions and cross references for the drugs. A new format allows dramatically improved readability and easier access to the information you need now.

Book • $99.50

Hardcover book, 12.5 x 9.5", 3533 pages, $99.50

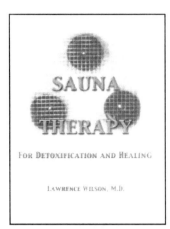

Book • $22.95

Sauna Therapy for Detoxification and Healing

By Lawrence Wilson, MD

This book provides a thorough yet articulate education on sauna therapy. It includes construction plans for a low-cost electric light sauna. The book is well referenced with an extensive bibliography.

Sauna therapy, especially with an electric light sauna, is one of the most powerful, safe and cost-effective methods of natural healing. It is especially important today due to extensive exposure to toxic metals and chemicals.

Fifteen chapters cover sauna benefits, physiological effects, protocols, cautions, healing reactions, and many other aspects of sauna therapy.

Dr. Wilson is an instructor of Biochemistry, Hair Mineral Analysis, Sauna Therapy and Jurisprudence at various colleges and universities including Yamuni Institute of the Healing Arts (Maurice, LA), University of Natural Medicine (Santa Fe, NM), Natural Healers Academy (Morristown, NJ), and Westbrook University (West Virginia). His books are used as textbooks at East-West School of Herbology and Ohio College of Natural Health. Go to www.LymeBook.com for free book excerpts!

Paperback book, 8.5 x 11", 167 pages, $22.95

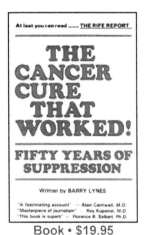

Book • $19.95

Over 50,000 Copies Sold!

The Cancer Cure That Worked: Fifty Years of Suppression

At Last You Can Read... The Rife Report

By Barry Lynes

Investigative journalism at its best. Barry Lynes takes readers on an exciting journey into the life work of Royal Rife. We are now the official publisher of this book. Call or visit us online for wholesale terms.

"A fascinating account..."
-Alan Cantwell, MD

"This book is superb."
-Florence B. Seibert, PhD

"Barry Lynes is one of the greatest health reporters in our country. With the assistance of John Crane, longtime friend and associate of Roy Rife, Barry has produced a masterpiece..." **-Roy Kupsinel, M.D., editor of *Health Consciousness Journal***

Paperback book, 5 x 8", 169 pages, $19.95

Rife Video Documentary
2-DVD Set, Produced by
Zero Zero Two Productions

Must-Have DVD set for your Rife technology education!

In 1999, a stack of forgotten audio tapes was discovered. On the tapes were the voices of several people at the center of the events which are the subject of this documentary: a revolutionary treatment for cancer and a practical cure for infectious disease.

The audio tapes were over 40 years old. The voices on them had almost faded, nearly losing key details of perhaps the most important medical story of the 20th Century.

But due to the efforts of the Kinnaman Foundation, the faded tapes have been restored and the voices on them recovered. So now, even though the participants have all passed away...

...they can finally tell their story.

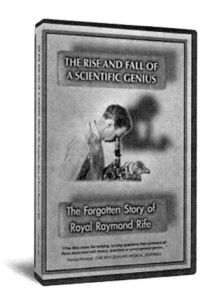

2-DVD Set • $39.95

"These videos are great. We show them at the Annual Rife International Health Conference."
-Richard Loyd, Ph.D.

"A mind-shifting experience for those of us indoctrinated with a conventional view of biology."
-Townsend Letter for Doctors and Patients

In the summer of 1934 at a special medical clinic in La Jolla, California, sixteen patients withering from terminal disease were given a new lease on life. It was the first controlled application of a new electronic treatment for cancer: the Beam Ray Machine.

Within ninety days all sixteen patients walked away from the clinic, signed-off by the attending doctors as cured.

What followed the incredible success of this revolutionary treatment was not a welcoming by the scientific community, but a sad tale of its ultimate suppression.

The Rise and Fall of a Scientific Genius documents the scientific ignorance, official corruption, and personal greed directed at the inventor of the Beam Ray Machine, Royal Raymond Rife, forcing him and his inventions out of the spotlight and into obscurity. **Just converted from VHS to DVD and completely updated.**

Includes bonus DVD with interviews and historical photographs! Produced in Canada.

Visit our website today to watch a FREE PREVIEW CLIP!

2 DVD-set, including bonus DVD, $39.95

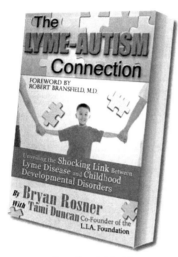

Book • $25.95

The Lyme-Autism Connection: Unveiling the Shocking Link Between Lyme Disease and Childhood Developmental Disorders

By Bryan Rosner & Tami Duncan

Did you know that Lyme disease may contribute to the onset of autism?

This book is an investigative report written by Bryan Rosner and Tami Duncan. Duncan is the co-founder of the *Lyme Induced Autism (LIA) Foundation*, and her son has an autism diagnosis.

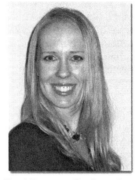

Tami Duncan, Co-Founder of the Lyme Induced Autism (LIA) Foundation

Awareness of the Lyme-autism connection is spreading rapidly, among both parents and practitioners. *Medical Hypothesis*, a scientific, peer-reviewed journal published by Elsevier, recently released an influential study entitled *The Association Between Tick-Borne Infections, Lyme Borreliosis and Autism Spectrum Disorders*. Here is an excerpt from the study:

> "Chronic infectious diseases, including tick-borne infections such as Borrelia burgdorferi, may have direct effects, promote other infections, and create a weakened, sensitized and immunologically vulnerable state during fetal development and infancy, leading to increased vulnerability for developing autism spectrum disorders. An association between Lyme disease and other tick-borne infections and autistic symptoms has been noted by numerous clinicians and parents."

—Medical Hypothesis Journal.
Article Authors: Robert C. Bransfield, M.D., Jeffrey S. Wulfman, M.D.,
William T. Harvey, M.D., Anju I. Usman, M.D.

Nationwide, 1 out of 150 children are diagnosed with Autism Spectrum Disorder (ASD), and the LIA Foundation has discovered that many of these children test positive for Lyme disease/Borrelia related complex—yet most children in this scenario never receive appropriate medical attention. This book answers many difficult questions: How can infants contract Lyme disease if autism begins before birth, precluding the opportunity for a tick bite? Is there a statistical correlation between the incidences of Lyme disease and autism worldwide? Do autistic children respond to Lyme disease treatment? What does the medical community say about this connection? Do the mothers of affected children exhibit symptoms? **Find out in this book.**

LIA FOUNDATION

Paperback book, 6x9", 287 pages, $25.95

Dietrich Klinghardt, M.D., Ph.D.
"Fundamental Teachings"
5-DVD Set

Includes Disc Exclusively For Lyme Disease!

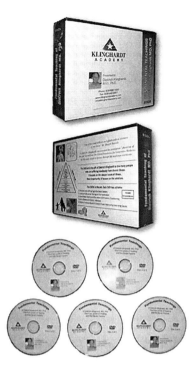

Dietrich Klinghardt, M.D., Ph.D. is a legendary healer known for discovering and refining many of the cutting-edge treatment protocols used for a variety of chronic health problems including Lyme disease, autism and mercury poisoning.

Now you can find out all about this doctor's treatment methods from the privacy of your own home! This 5-DVD set includes the following DVDs:

- **DISC 1**: The Five Levels of Healing and the Seven Factors

- **DISC 2**: Autonomic Response Testing and Demonstration

- **DISC 3**: Heavy Metal Toxicity and Neurotoxin Elimination / Electrosmog

- **DISC 4:** Lyme disease and Chronic Illness

- **DISC 5**: Psycho-Emotional Issues in Chronic Illness & Addressing Underlying Causes

5-DVD Set • $125

Dr. Dietrich Klinghardt is one of the most important contributors to modern integrative treatment for Lyme disease and related medical conditions. This comprehensive DVD set is a must-have addition to your educational library.

5-DVD Set, $125

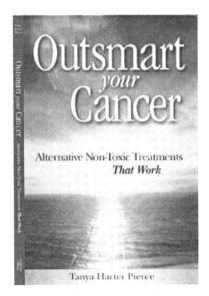

Book and Audio CD • $24.50

Outsmart Your Cancer: Alternative Non-Toxic Treatments That Work   By Tanya Harter Pierce

Why BLUDGEON cancer to death with common conventional treatments that can be toxic and harmful to your entire body?

When you OUTSMART your cancer, only the cancer cells die — NOT your healthy cells! *OUTSMART YOUR CANCER: Alternative Non-Toxic Treatments That Work* is an easy guide to successful non-toxic treatments for cancer that you can obtain right now! In it, you will read real-life stories of people who have completely recovered from their advanced or late-stage lung cancer, breast cancer, prostate cancer, kidney cancer, brain cancer, childhood leukemia, and other types of cancer using effective non-toxic approaches.

Plus, *OUTSMART YOUR CANCER* is one of the few books in print today that gives a complete description of the amazing formula called "Protocel," which has produced incredible cancer recoveries over the past 20 years. **A supporting audio CD is included with this book**. Pricing = $19.95 book + $5.00 CD.

Paperback book, 6 x 9", 437 pages, with audio CD, $24.95

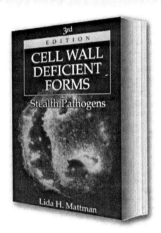

Hardcover Book • $169.95

Cell Wall Deficient Forms: Stealth Pathogens

By Lida Mattman, Ph.D.

This is one of the most influential infectious disease textbook of the century. Dr. Mattman, who earned a Ph.D. in immunology from Yale University, describes her discovery that a certain type of pathogen lacking a cell wall is the root cause of many of today's "incurable" and mysterious chronic diseases. Dr. Mattman's research is the foundation of our current understanding of Lyme disease, and her work led to many of the Lyme protocols used today (such as the Marshall Protocol, as well as modern LLMD antibiotic treatment strategy). Color illustrations and meticulously referenced breakthrough principles cover the pages of this book. A must have for all serious students of chronic, elusive infectious disease.

Hardcover book, 7.5 x 10.5", 416 pages, $169.95

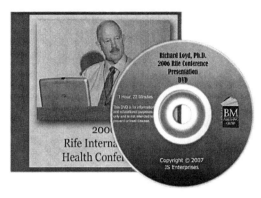

DVD • $24.50

Richard Loyd, Ph.D., presents at the Rife International Health Conference in Seattle

Watch this DVD to gain a better understanding of the technical details of rife technology.

Dr. Loyd, who earned a Ph.D. in nutrition, has researched and experimented with numerous electrotherapeutic devices, including the Rife/Bare unit, various EMEM machines, F-Scan, BioRay, magnetic pulsers, Doug Machine, and more. Dr. Loyd also has a wealth of knowledge in the use of herbs and supplements to support Rife electromagnetics.

By watching this DVD, you will discover the nuts and bolts of some very important, yet little known, principles of rife machine operation, including:

- Gating, sweeping, session time
- Square vs. sine wave
- DC vs. AC frequencies
- Duty cycle
- Octaves and scalar octaves

- Voltage variations and radio frequencies
- Explanation of the spark gap
- Contact vs. radiant mode
- Stainless vs. copper contacts
- A unique look at various frequency devices

DVD, 57 minutes, $24.50

Under Our Skin:
Lyme Disease Documentary Film

A gripping tale of microbes, medicine & money, UNDER OUR SKIN exposes the hidden story of Lyme disease, one of the most serious and controversial epidemics of our time. Each year, thousands go undiagnosed or misdiagnosed, often told that their symptoms are all in their head. Following the stories of patients and physicians fighting for their lives and livelihoods, the film brings into focus a haunting picture of the health care system and a medical establishment all too willing to put profits ahead of patients.

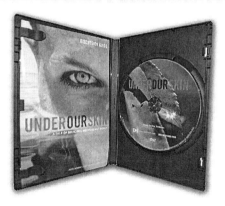

DVD • $34.95

Bonus Features: 32-page discussion guidebook, one hour of bonus footage, director's commentary, and much more! **FOR HOME USE ONLY**

DVD with bonus features, 104 minutes, $34.95 *MUST SEE!*

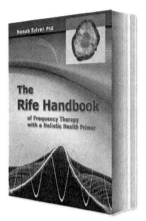

Book • $112.50

The Rife Handbook of Frequency Therapy, With a Holistic Health Primer

Revised 2011 Edition! By Nenah Sylver, PhD

This is the most complete, authoritative Rife technology handbook in the world. A hardcover book, it weighs over 2 lbs. and has more than 730 pages. A broad range of practical, hands-on topics are covered:

- New Revised Edition released in 2011 is twice as long as original book! Now with a complete index!
- Royal Raymond Rife's life, inventions, and relationships.
- Recently discovered data explaining how Rife's original machines worked.
- Frequently Asked Questions about Rife sessions and equipment, with extensive session information.
- Ground-breaking information on strengthening and supporting the body.
- A 200-page, cross-referenced Frequency Directory including hundreds of health conditions.
- Bibliography, Three Appendices, Historical Photos, Complete Index, AND MUCH MORE!
- DVD available at www.LymeBook.com with author's recent Rife Conference presentation.

Hardcover book, 8.5 x 11", 730 pages, $112.50

Index

5-HTP 148-9
5-methyl-tetra-hydro-folate 148, 152
5-methyl-tetrahdro-folate 175
24-hour saliva cortisol test 13
24-hour urine collection 96

A

Acidophilus 130
Additives 9, 12, 30-1, 41, 44, 155
ADHD 61, 94
Adjustments, osteopathic 182
Adrenal fatigue 1-9, 12-17, 21, 50, 148, 200, 215
Adrenal glands 1-4, 6-19, 39, 42, 47, 151, 182-3, 203
Adrenaline 1, 4, 18
Aflatoxins 78-9
Air conditioners 71, 82
Alcohol 2, 42, 155, 163
Allergies 27, 34, 37-8, 52, 81, 115-16, 134, 155, 160, 189-90
Aloe vera 128, 164
Alpha-lipoic acid 106, 108
Alzheimer's disease 135, 150
Amalgams 61-2, 70, 168, 176, 181
Amino acids 10, 20, 42, 128, 147-50, 152
Amoebas 114
Amoxicillin 195
Amylase breaks 128
Anaplasmosis 189, 201
Andrew Hall Cutler 220-1, 225
Anemia 96, 99, 115, 152
Anger 137, 140-1, 144
Animal protein 12, 33, 35, 38, 42, 44, 150
Anorexia nervosa 190
Antennas 61-2, 67, 69, 85
Anti-anxiety treatments 212
Anti-parasitic remedies 111
Antibiotics 23, 28, 32, 37, 40-1, 44, 51, 58, 123-7, 129, 131-2, 161-2, 167, 195-6, 202-3
 cyst-busting 196
 toxic 195
Antibodies 75, 79, 89, 165, 193
Antibody tests 19, 198, 211
Antidepressants 156
Antidiuretic hormone 90

Antifungal treatments 160, 162
Antimicrobial herbs 167
Antioxidants 10, 48, 99, 150, 202
Anxiety 2, 5, 9, 61, 86, 93-4, 137-8, 150, 155-6, 190, 192, 197, 210, 212
Appetite 96, 99, 153, 208
Apple pectin 176
Appliances, household 53, 65, 67, 71-2
Applied kinesiology 101, 104, 116-18
Artemisia 121, 199, 207
Arthralgia 197, 201
Arthritis 27, 100, 172, 191, 204
Artichoke 39
Artificial sweeteners 40, 163
Ascorbic acid 9, 48
Ascorbyl palmitate 48
Ashwagandha 8
Asthma 134, 208
ASYRA 197
Atovaquone 198, 209
Austria 56-7
Autism 94, 111, 173, 177
Autoimmune diseases 27, 29, 52, 125, 168, 171-4, 184
Autoimmunity 54, 88
Autonomic nervous system (ANS) 1, 178-9, 181, 189-90, 200
Ayurvedic herb 119
Azithromycin 195, 198, 201

B

B-vitamins (see also Vitamin B) 50, 130, 152, 175
Babesia 6, 48, 114, 149, 164-5, 167, 188-90, 195, 197-9, 201, 207-12
Baby monitors 69
Baltimore 219
Banderol 83, 85, 197, 220
Barley 34, 131
Barron, Jon 123-4, 130
Bartonella 6, 114, 188-9, 197-8, 201, 208, 210-12, 214, 225
Baseline of Health Foundation 222
Beans 38, 150, 155
Becker, Robert 54
Bed 64-6, 69
Bed sheets 66, 69-70

Bedroom 65, 82
Bee propolis 81
Beef 27, 37, 151
   grass-fed 47
   uncooked 120
Beets 39, 175
Belgium 57
Beliefs 11, 136-7, 142, 144-5, 223
   harmful 141
   healthier 139, 158
   unhealthy 136-7, 139-40, 147
Bentonite clay 84
BHT 30
Bifidobacteria 130
Bile 84, 106, 128
Binders 85, 106, 108, 176
Bioenergetic medicine 101, 118, 197-8
Biofilms 137, 148, 161, 164, 166, 188, 196, 200, 202
Bioidentical hormones 147, 157-8
Bioidentical T3 hormone 16, 20
BioMed Publishing Group 178, 225-6
Biophoton treatments 62, 126
BioPure 49, 102
Biosynthesis 90
Biotech firms 26
Biotin 49, 94, 96, 99
Biotoxins 75, 79, 173, 180, 216
Bisphenol-A (BPA) 30
Black-eyed peas 38
Black walnut 119, 121
Bladder 213
Bland, Jeffrey 11
Blastocystis hominis 114
Bloating 28-9, 115-16, 153, 160
Blood 1, 18-20, 46, 60, 90, 98, 165, 168, 209
Blood brain barrier 59, 108
Blood cell mineral test, red 104
Blood sugar imbalances 1, 12, 40, 127
Blood sugar spikes 35, 38-9
Blood vessels 48, 171, 190, 213
Bluetooth wireless headsets 63-4
Blurred vision 88
Bock, Steven 14
Bok choy 39
Boluoke 166
Bone 99, 169-70, 172-3, 179, 181
Borrelia 6, 14, 113-14, 126, 134, 148, 164-7, 173, 179, 181, 187-96, 210

Borrelia cysts 166
Boundaries, healthy relational 6-7, 146, 223
Bowthorpe, Janie 16, 18, 215
BPA (Bisphenol-A) 30
Brain 46-7, 60-1, 106, 108, 112, 115, 138, 140, 146-7, 150, 155-6, 179, 192
Brain cancer 60, 64, 155
Brain fog 5, 19, 46, 116, 138
Brazil nuts 38
Bread 34, 36
Breast 29-31
Breast milk 203
Brittle hair 99
Broccoli 25, 39
Brucella 190, 201
Brussels sprouts 39
Bulbs 69
   fluorescent light 69
   incandescent 69
Burrascano, Joseph 187, 196
Butyrate 121, 132
Butyric acid 129

C

Cabbage 39
Caffeine 2, 12, 42-3, 155, 163
Calcium 25, 41, 49, 149
Canada 24, 216, 224
Cancer 27, 29-31, 41, 52, 54-6, 59-61, 79, 94, 111, 135, 157, 168, 172-4, 218
Candida 53, 159-64, 184, 224
Canned food products 30
Caprylic acid 162
Carbohydrates 12, 23, 36, 100, 126, 128, 160
Carcinogens 23, 69
Cardiac problems 9, 50
Caregivers 136, 145
Carlo, George 55, 61
Carpet 82, 174
Carrageenan 30, 32, 41, 131
Carrots 39, 175
Cavitations 168-71, 173
CD-57 test 191, 194, 208
CDC *see* Centers for Disease Control
Ceftin 195
Celery 39, 175
Cell membranes 61, 180
Cell phone 53-5, 63-5, 68, 71-2, 86

Cell phone antenna 63
Cell phone base station 63
Cell phone dangers 55
Cell phone network 65
Cell phone signal 63
Centers for Disease Control (CDC) 153, 177, 188, 191-3
Central nervous system (CNS) 60, 115, 156, 179, 192
Ceramic tile 82
Cheese 32, 41, 85, 155
Chelation Therapy 106-8, 221
Chemical burn 213
Chemicals 30, 32, 44, 151, 155, 173-4, 189
Chicken 37
    free-range 47, 150
Chicken bones 10
Chicken broth, prepared 10-11
Chills 197, 208
China 56
Chinese medicine 14
Chiropractic 178-9, 182
Chlamydia 165, 189, 200-1
Chlorella 106, 108, 131, 176
Chlorine 51, 124
Chlorine dioxide 83
Chlorox 176
Chocolate 43, 131, 155
Cholestepure 84, 220
Cholestyramine 84, 90, 220
Christmas 43
Chromium 49, 94
Chromosomes 27
Chronic fatigue syndrome 1, 3, 15, 95, 115, 141, 145, 154, 173, 191, 201
Chronic Lyme disease 2, 4, 6, 11, 19, 48-9, 58, 91, 95, 161, 164-5, 173, 188-9, 191-2, 203-4
Chronic sinus infection 91, 160
Chronic vaginal yeast infections 160
Churches 143
Cilantro 106, 108
Cinnamon 43, 81, 83
Ciprofloxin 195
Circuit breakers 65
Circulation problems 190
CIRS-WDB 87-91
Citric acid 83
Cleocin 199

Clindamycin 209
Clongen 197
Cloud, Henry 146
Clove bud oil 197
Clove oil 119
Cloves 81, 83, 121
CMV 190
Co-infections 14, 48, 134, 167, 189, 192, 200-1
Coartem 199
Coated tongue 160
Coconut 39, 41
Coconut kefir 131
Coconut milk 41
Coconut oil 12, 176
Cod liver oil 181
Coffee 42-3, 78
Coffee enemas 175
Colitis 115-16
Collagen 48, 181, 188
Colon 129, 155
Colostrum 134, 163-4
Computer 55, 60, 64, 66, 70-2, 86
Computer screen 70
Concentration problems 60, 77
Confusion 8, 45-6, 77, 88, 102
Conjugated linoleic acid 29
Conjunctivitis 99
Constipation 96, 115, 153, 155
Copper 97, 102, 104-5
CoQ10 151
Cordain, Loren 44
CORE product 49, 103, 216
Corn 9, 28-9, 155, 163, 204
Cortisol 4, 11, 13, 16-20, 42, 157, 215
Costa Rica 83
Cottage cheese 149
Counselors 138, 141-2, 144
Cow 27-30, 40, 131
Cow acidosis 29
Cow dairy products 40
Cowden, Lee 81, 126, 146, 174-5, 187, 222
Cow's stomach compartments 28
Coxsackie virus 165, 201
Cramps 45, 50
Cranial sacral manipulation 180
Cravings 42
    salt 2
Creatine monohydrate 152, 175

Criminal Behavior 220
Crock-Pot 36
Cryptolepsis 199
Cucumbers 39, 175
Cumanda 83, 197
Cummins, Joe 27
Custom Probiotics Inc 130, 222
Cyanocobalamin (*see also* Vitamin B-12) 154
Cytokine response 76, 83, 135
Cytomegalovirus 165

D

Dairy 9, 34-5, 40-1, 44, 131, 155, 163, 204, 216
   pasteurized 12
Dairy kefir products 131
Dairy products
   commercial 40, 131
   goat's 131
   unpasteurized 40
Dallas 216, 226
Davis, Anne 5, 13
DEET 210, 214
Deficiencies 18, 20, 24, 45, 47, 49-52, 94, 99-102, 104, 156
   biotin 99-100
   common 45
   enzyme 190
   estrogen 157
   hormone 42
   hydrochloric acid 35
   immune 116
   molybdenum 100
   neurotransmitter 99, 147
Dehydration 61
Denmark 56
Dentists 169-71, 177
   biological 170-2, 176
Denver 67, 154
Depression 2, 19, 43, 45-6, 49-50, 60-1, 93-5, 99, 133-5, 137-41, 145-51, 153, 155-8, 197-8, 212
Dermatitis 99-100
Desserts 43
   gluten-free 43
Detoxification 1, 5-6, 10, 13-14, 43, 48, 66, 81-2, 97-8, 100, 105, 173-7, 199-200, 202, 216
Dextrose 181

DHA 150
Diabetes 39, 100, 135, 223
Diarrhea 29, 88, 115, 153, 155
Diffuser, cold air 80-1
Diflucan 161-2
Digestion 12, 27, 32, 34-6, 40-1, 60, 115, 124, 127-9, 222
DMPS 106-8, 176
DMSA 106-8, 176
DNA 24, 27, 53, 59, 79, 136, 151-2, 165, 174, 176, 188-9, 193
   extracellular 166
   foreign 27
   interspecies 166
DNP 45
Dopamine 147-8, 150
Doxycycline 195, 197, 201
Dust 79-80, 87

E

Earthing 66-7, 217, 219
EAV/EDS-type biofeedback devices 104, 117
EBay 63, 69
EDTA 107
EFAs (Essential Fatty Acids) 46
Egg protein powder 44
Egg yolks 155
Eggs 47, 150, 155, 204
Ehrlichia 164, 189, 201, 209
Eicosapentaenoic acid 150
Electrical conductivity 117
Electro-acupuncture 117
Electrodermal screening 117
Electromagnetic fields 53-61, 63, 65-7, 69, 71-3, 85-6, 126, 173, 181, 217-18
Electrons 66
ELISA test 192-3
EMF Safety Store 69-70, 219
Emotional stressor 140
Emotional trauma 4, 133-7, 139-43, 145-9, 151, 153, 155, 157-8, 200, 223
Emotional well-being 103
Emotions 146, 155-6
Encephalitis 201
Endocrine abnormalities 190
Endotoxins 86
Enlarged livers 28, 209
Enlarged lymph nodes 210
Enlarged spleen 209

Enzymes 32, 35, 40-1, 90, 124, 127-9, 131-2, 151, 156, 173
Eosinophils 208
EPA 150
Epsom salt baths 175
Epstein-Barr 165
Equilibrium 199
Erwin, Vernon 168, 225
Erythropoietin 88
Esophagus 155
Essential oils 80-1, 210, 214
Estradiol 156
Estrogen 40, 156-7, 224
EVOX system 146
Exercises 175, 182, 184, 190, 203, 207
    aerobic 203
    core-strengthening 183

F

Faraday cage 64-6, 69
Fatigue 2-3, 5, 8-9, 19, 36, 45, 50, 60, 77, 88, 100, 115-16, 120, 197, 207-8
Fats 9, 12, 39, 42, 50, 100, 126, 128
Fecal matter 114, 120
Fermented Asian tea 131
Fermented dairy product 130
Fermented foods 40, 161
Fermented Korean dish, traditional 130
Fertility 100
Fever 201, 208, 210
    spotted 201, 209
Fiber 35, 129
Fibroblasts 181
Fibromyalgia 3, 15, 95, 115, 173, 191
Fingernails 95
Fish 28, 33, 37-8, 47, 150-1, 155, 198
FISH test 198
Flagyl 166
Floradix 49
Folic acid 152, 154
Food additives 30
Food allergies 2, 30, 34, 36-7, 44, 76, 96, 115, 204, 224
Food-based iron products 49, 100
Forgiveness 139-41, 144
Formaldehyde 174
Forsgren, Scott 48
Free T3 levels 15, 19
French Association for Research in Therapeutics 61, 218

Frozen foods 31
Fruits 25, 33, 35, 38, 44, 78, 163
    colored 150
    high-glycemic 38, 85
    low-glycemic 35
    non-starchy 44
Fukushima 174, 176
Fungal infections 42, 75, 78, 83, 124, 129, 131, 159-62, 164, 189, 202
Fungicides 124, 132

G

Gall bladder 84, 128, 175
Gaussmeter 65, 67-9
Gene expression 50, 151
Gentian root 119
Giardia 114, 120
Gilber, Gloria 124
Gilham, Peter 45
Ginger root 119
Gingivitis 212
Glaros, William 170, 225
Gluconeogenesis 50
Glucose 42, 50, 100, 127
Glutathione 10, 107-8, 176
Gluten 34-5, 43, 90, 155, 163, 204
Glycoproteins 188
GMOs (Genetically modified organisms) 26-8, 30-1, 44, 48, 52, 54, 132-3, 155
Goat's milk cheese 40-1
God 23, 139
Goldenseal root 119
Golf courses 210, 214
Grains 12, 29, 31, 33-6, 38, 44, 78, 85, 124, 155, 204
Granola bars 31-2
Grapefruit 38, 162-3
Great Britain 27

H

Hamstring 161
Hartman, Stan 62, 67-8, 219
Headaches 50, 60, 76-7, 88, 100, 153, 192, 197, 201, 207
Headsets, wired 63-4
Heat 130
Heavy metal binders 85, 108, 176
Heavy metals 47-8, 51-2, 61-2, 70, 85-6, 93-5, 97-8, 103, 105-9, 120, 173-4, 177, 200

Heel 175
Helicobacter pylori 201
Heme 93
Hemochromatosis 105
Hemoglobin 49-50, 93
Hemolytic anemia 209
Hemopyrrollactamuria 93
Hemp 44, 150
HEPA 82
Herbicides 30-2, 52, 124, 132
Herpes 165
Herxheimer reactions 5, 81, 118, 138, 144, 199, 207
HHV-6 190
HHV-8 190
High-velocity manipulation 180
Hips 183
Hoffer, Abram 93
Homeopathics 20, 117, 146, 170, 175
Homeostasis 11, 199
Homocysteine 153
Hookworms 112, 114
Hormones 6, 10-11, 13, 15-16, 18, 20, 23, 29-30, 40-2, 44-5, 90-1, 127, 147, 157, 173-4
Horowitz, Richard 189, 196, 198
Hot flashes 208
Houttuynia 197
Huggins, Hal 168, 171, 225
Humaworm 121, 221
Hydrochloric acid 127, 132
Hydrocortisone 11, 18-19
Hyperactivity 99
Hypercoagulation 46
Hypochlorhydria 102
Hypoglycemia 2, 5, 12, 38-9, 96, 115
Hypotension 2
Hypothalamus 91
Hypothyroidism 1, 3, 5, 7, 9, 11, 13, 15-17, 19-21, 215

I

Ice-cream 179
IDSA (Infectious Diseases Society of America) 192, 204
IgeneX 193, 197
IGF-1 29
IL-6 88
ILADS (International Lyme and Associated Diseases Society) 160-1, 166, 187, 196,

199, 202, 204, 224
Immune complexes 193
Immune modulators 134
Immune suppression 11, 106, 111, 145, 158, 160
Impatience 213
Incandescent lightbulbs 56
India 150
Infertility 31
Infrared saunas 175
Ingredients 32-3, 35, 43
    all natural 31
    artificial 52
Insecticides 124
Insomnia 2, 9, 19, 45-6, 60, 95, 99, 126, 192, 197, 200-1, 207-8, 210, 212
Insulin 29, 38-9, 127, 190, 217
Iodine 17, 20, 49, 174
Iodoquinol 119
Ionic footbaths 84
Iron 20, 48-9, 93, 100, 104-5, 149, 162
Irritability 2, 9, 45-6, 94, 96, 99, 138, 190, 197, 212-13
Irritable bowel syndrome 2, 29, 41, 115, 123, 155
Itching 76, 213
IV Claforan 195
IV Rocephin 195
IV therapy 200
IV vancomycin 195
Ivermectin 119
IVIG 200

J

Jaundice 100, 209
Jawbone 169, 172-3
Jones, Bob 169
Jordan Rubin 23, 35
Journal of Orthomolecular Medicine 93, 220

K

Kale 39
Kane, Patricia 44, 216
Kansas City 216
Kefir 41, 130-1
Kidneys 98, 100, 175, 177
Kombucha 41, 131

KPU (Also known as Pyroluria) 93-6, 220-1
Kunold, Marlene 14

L

L-cysteine 149
L-cystine 149
L-glutamine 121, 128-9
L-phenylalaline 148, 150
L-tryptophan 148-50
L-tyrosine 17, 148, 150
Lab Corp 47
Lab tests 12-13, 78, 80, 88-9, 97, 112, 116, 153, 197-8, 208-9, 211-12
Lab Tests for Babesia 198
Lab Tests for Bartonella 197
Lab Tests for Borrelia 192
Laguna Beach 217
Lake Tahoe 225-6
Lam, Michael 3, 215
Lancet 29
Larium 207-8
Leaky gut syndrome 31, 41, 45, 123-4, 222
Legacy Line Publishing 225
Legumes 38, 163
Lemon juice 38, 81, 83, 85
Lentils 38, 150
Lesions 46, 112, 170
Lettuce 39
Leukaemia 59, 218
Leukemia 31, 69
Leukopenia 201
Levaquin 195, 197
Levofloxacin 201
Libido 2, 192
Licorice 8
Life events, stressful 155
Life Extension Magazine 25, 55, 217-18
Lifestyle modifications 7-8, 21, 124, 142, 211
Ligament laxity 100, 180, 183-4
Ligament tissue, new 181
Ligaments, damaged 179
Light sensitivity 77, 88
Lincoln University 55, 218
Lipids 48, 100, 188
Liposomal Glutathione 10
Liposomal nutrients 9, 48
Lipton, Bruce 136
Liver 79, 98, 100, 115, 155, 175, 177

Livestock 28-9, 31, 33, 41
Lugol's iodine solution 174
Lupus 191
Lymph vessels 168
Lymphatic drainage obstruction 182
Lymphoma 218

M

Macrolide 195, 199, 201
Macular degeneration 99
Magnesium 45, 49, 148, 152, 184
Maker's Diet 35
Malarone 198-9
Manganese 49, 94, 100, 102, 104
Marshmallow 121, 128-9, 132, 164, 175
Mayo Clinic 172
MCIDS (Multiple Chronic Infectious Disease Syndrome) 189
Mebendazole 119
Melanocyte-stimulating hormone (MSH) 88, 91
Memory 45, 96, 210, 223
Memory problems 46, 60, 77, 88, 192, 197, 210
Meningitis 201, 204
Menstrual cycle 2, 95, 192
Mental clarity 100
Mental confusion 153
Mental hospitals 93
Mental imagery 183
Mental performance 112, 221
Mepron 198-9, 207
Mercola, Joseph 28, 63, 124, 176, 217-18, 222
Mercury 37-8, 47, 106-8, 150, 168, 173, 176-7, 220
Metabolism 15, 18, 42, 50, 100, 151
Metal furniture 66, 69-70
Methionine 152-3
Methyl donors 151-2
Methyl groups 151
Methylation 97, 148, 151-2
Methylation tests 152
Methylcobalamin (see also: Vitamin B-12) 154
Methylmalonic acid 153
Metronidazole 119, 195-6
Microwaves 60, 65, 69
Milk 29, 41
   almond 32

animal's 203
  homemade nut 43
  nondairy 32
  sheep's 41
Milk thistle 175
Milligauss 57, 68
Mimosa pudica 119
Mineral deficiencies 49, 51, 97-8, 101, 120
Minocycline 195
Miracle Mineral Supplement 83
Misalignments, vertebral 177-80, 182
Moisture 80, 130
Moles 213
Molybdenum 49, 94, 100
Monosodium glutamate 30
Monsanto 26
Mood disorders 192
Mood regulation 147, 151
Morning stiffness 88
Mortality 55, 59, 218
MSH (melanocyte-stimulating hormone) 88, 91
Mucopolysaccharide matrix 166
Mucuna bean powder 150
Multiple chemical sensitivities 2, 189
Muscle aches 45, 115, 209
Muscle contraction 45
Muscle cramps 77, 88
Muscle/joint pain 60
Muscle strength 183
Muscle twitches 46
Muscle weakness 50, 61, 99, 197
Muscles 104, 115-17, 183-4, 192
  arm 117
  sore 192
Musculoskeletal problems 182, 184, 192
Mustard greens 39
Musty smell 79, 82-3
Myalgic encephalomyelitis 141
Mycoplasma 164, 189, 194, 200-1
Mycotoxins 59, 75-9, 81, 83, 85-7, 89, 91, 219
Myelin 151, 180, 184
Myhill, Sarah 141, 223

N

N-acetyl-cysteine 166
Nagy, Lisa 76
National Cancer Institute 29, 55, 217
National Institutes of Health (NIH) 204

Nattokinase 166
Natural bug spray 31
Natural Calm products 45
Natural flavoring 30
Natural food products 32
Natural killer (NK) cells 134
Nausea 50, 60, 100, 153, 155, 201, 209
Nerve conduction 45
Nerve damage 180
Nerves 168, 171, 179-80, 184, 192, 200
Nervous system 4, 61, 155, 178-80, 184, 190, 192
Nervousness 2, 115
Neuroendocrine problems 1, 91
Neurotoxins 13
Neurotransmitters 42, 99, 147-8, 150-2, 155
New York Times 28, 33, 217
New Zealand 46
NIH (National Institutes of Health) 204
Nikken air filters 82, 220
Nitazoxanide 119
Nobel Prize 54
Non-gluten grains 36, 38, 44, 155
Non-Hodgkin's lymphoma 31
Non-metal-containing mattress 66
Non-organic milk products 29
Nordic Naturals 47, 151
Numbness 50, 61, 77, 88, 99
Nut butters 38, 85
NutraMedix 83, 166, 175, 187, 196, 220
Nutrient absorption 99, 124, 130, 156
Nutrient assimilation 124
Nuts 12, 35, 38, 46, 85, 150
  allergenic 163
  pine 38
Nystatin 161-2

O

Oats 31, 34-5
Ochratoxins 78
Olive leaf extract 83
Omega-3 EFAs 38, 46-7, 150-1
Omega-6 EFAs 29, 38, 46
Omnicef 195
Onions 39
Oregano 162

Oxygen 46, 153, 183
Ozone 81, 181
Ozone air purifiers 81
Ozone generators 81

P

P-5-P 149
Pain 5, 60, 77, 88, 95, 115, 134, 138, 141, 143, 147, 169, 179-80, 182-3, 200
    abdominal 50, 77, 88
    back/hip/pelvic 183-4
    emotional 138
    eye 197
    ice-pick-like 88
    joint 77, 88, 96, 100, 181, 197, 201
    musculoskeletal 2, 99, 197
    neck 169
    neuropathic 192
    soft tissue 201
Paleo Diet Cookbook 44
Pancreas 127-8
Pantethine 10, 17
Pantothenic acid 10, 17, 50
Paranoia 96, 153, 190
Parasite cleanses 112-13, 118, 121
Parastroy 121, 221
Paresthesia 50
Parkinson's disease 61, 100, 150, 152, 173, 177, 191
Parsley 108, 175
Pasteurization 32, 40, 131
PCR test 193
Peanut butter 85
Peanuts 38, 85, 155, 163, 204
Pecans 38, 43
Pekana 175
Pelvis 183
Penicillins 195
Perfectionism 3, 6-7, 145
Periods
    extended 18, 37, 66
    short 67
Pernicious anemia 154
Pesticides, chemical 23, 25, 31
Petaluma 220
PH 29, 48
Phagocytosis 129
Pharmacies, compounding 21, 49, 154
Phenol glycerine 181
Phone 63-4

cordless 53, 56, 58, 63, 68
    mobile 58
    speaker 64
Phos-Chol 180
Phosphatidyl-choline 180
Phospholipids 152
Phthalates 157
Physical therapists 183
Pilates 144, 182-4, 203, 224
Pinella 175
Pinworms 114, 190
Plastic beverage bottles 31
Plastic residue 31
Plastics 23, 30-1, 51, 157
Pneumonia 29, 201, 208
Poesnecker, Gerald 3, 5, 145, 215
Pollan, Michael 23, 28, 33, 216-17
Pollutants 51, 53-4, 73, 124, 133
    environmental 58, 134
    inorganic 51
Polypeptides 128
Polysaccharide matrixes 148
Polysaccharides 128
Porcine glands 21
Pork 37, 120
Posture 178, 183
Potassium bromate 30
Potassium iodide 176
Potato 25, 155, 163
    sweet 38
Potatoes, white 39
Prayer 140-1, 144
Praziquantel 119
Pregnancy 203
Prescript-Assist Pro 129, 222
Primaxin 195
Pro-inflammatory cytokines 88, 135
Probiotics 41, 75, 111, 121, 124, 129-32, 163, 222
Processed foods 12, 28, 40, 52, 123-4, 155
Processed Meat 28
Product labels 32
Progesterone 156-7
Progestins 157, 224
Prolotherapy 181, 183-4, 224
Prolozone 181
Protease 128
Protein 1, 10, 15, 30, 34, 38, 40, 44-5, 48, 50, 59, 90, 126, 135-6, 151-2
Protozoa 114, 200, 209, 211

Provera 157
Pumice 181
Pumpkin 38, 119, 149
Pyrental pamoate 119
Pyridoxal phosphate 50, 102, 149
Pyridoxine 99

Q

Quinoa 38, 44
Quinolone-type antibiotics 195, 201

R

Rabbit 172
Radiation 57, 62-4, 69-71, 176
   high-frequency 68, 70
   low-frequency 68, 71
   measuring radio/microwave 68
   radio frequency 65
Radioactive particles 176
Rage 96, 140, 192, 211-12
Rau, Thomas M. 58, 218
Raven Press 225
Raw dairy 40, 131
Raw vegetables 12, 35-6
Refrigerator 85
ReNew Life's ParaGone 121, 221
Researched Nutritionals 129-30, 163, 222
Reverse osmosis 51
Rice, brown 36, 38, 85
Rice bread 35
Rifampin 195, 197, 201
Rikettsia 189
Roberts, James 221
Root canals 168-9, 171-3, 225
Rosner, Bryan 178, 225
Roundworms 112, 114
Router, wireless Wi-Fi 62
Rye 34, 131

S

S-adenosyl methionine 152
Sahelian, Ray 135, 223
Salad 35-6
Saliva 79, 128
Saliva cortisol tests 13, 82, 202
Saliva sample 165
Salmon 37, 47, 150
Samento 166, 196-7
San Diego 225

Santa Rosa 223
Sardines 37, 47, 150
Sauerkraut 41, 130-1
Savely, Ginger 45
Scallions 39
Schaller, James 84, 91, 188, 197-8, 207, 209, 219, 225
Schatz, Linda 164, 224
Schizophrenia 93-5, 190, 220
Schwarzbein Principle 46, 216
Seizures 95, 197
Selenium 20, 49
Self-control 7
Septra 198
Serotonin 42, 99, 147-9, 151, 155-6
Sesame 38
Shoemaker, Ritchie 86-7, 89-91, 219
Siberian ginseng 8
Siegel, Bernie 135, 223
Sinatra, Stephen 107, 217
Singleton, Ken 150, 187, 216, 226
Sinus cavities 91
Sinus problems 77, 88
Skin 48, 51, 96, 114-15, 154, 171, 175, 209, 212-13
   dry 99
Skin rashes 61
Skin redness 76
Skin sensitivity 88
Sleep 2, 5, 8, 50, 64-6, 115, 183, 190, 208, 210, 212
Slippery elm 121, 128, 164
Smartphones 53-4
Smoked meats 85
Sneezing 76
Snow, David 194
Socioeconomic status 223
Sodium nitrate 30
Soft-tissue sarcomas 31
Soil 25, 32, 49, 114, 120-1, 130
   mineral-rich 33
   purify 129
Solvents 174
Soul 7, 34, 136-40, 143
   wounded 138
Soul sickness 138
Sounds/light 2
Soups 12, 35, 131
Soy 27-8, 30, 32, 40, 44, 46, 155, 163, 204, 217

Spinach 39
Spinal cord 178-9, 182-3, 192
Spiro Stat Technologies 194
Spirochetes 195, 203
Spiroplast 195
Spirulina 131, 176
Spores 78, 81, 85
Spouse 210, 214
Sprained ankle 180
St. John's Wort 156
Stachybotrys 78
Stamina 8, 138
Starch 28, 128-9
Steroid hormones 1, 11, 16-18, 90
Steroids 11, 18, 196
Stevia 39, 43
Stomach acid 12, 99, 102, 121
Stomach pain 155
Stool tests 116
Strokes 157
Strongyloides 190
Sublingual 154
Subluxations 177-8, 182-3
Substance abuse 135
Sugar 2, 38, 41-4, 124, 128, 131, 162-3, 181, 204
   artificial 160
   cane 131
   fruit juice 41
   low blood 2
   refined 9, 12, 41-2
Sulfa-type drugs 201
Sunflower 155
Surgery 169-71, 213
Sweats 77, 88, 197, 208
Sweetening beverages 43
Switzerland 56
Synthroid 20

T

T-cells 88, 193
T4 19
Tachycardia 100
Taheebo tea 163
Tapeworms 114, 120
Taylor, Julianne 46
Tea, green 43
Teeth 169-70, 172, 176
Teeth grinding 115
Teich, Morton 160-1, 224

Temperament 5
Temperature 20, 212
   basal 20
   body's morning 20
   low body 2, 15
Temperature-regulation problems 88
Tendon structures 100, 180
Tension 179
TERF (Toxic Element Research Foundation) 172
Tetracyclines 119, 195, 201
Texas 216
TGF B-1 88, 90
Thieves oil 80-1, 220
Thinking
   angry 8
   negative 139
Thoracic vertebra 178
Thoughts 136-40, 144, 147, 158
   healthy 149
   negative 136
   toxic 139
Thrombocytopenia 201
Thumb 32, 38
Thyroid 1, 6, 13, 15-21, 40, 47, 100, 157, 176, 215
Tick bite 188, 192, 210
Tigecycline 195-6
Tingling 50, 77, 88, 99
Tinidazole 119, 166, 195-6
TMJ 182
Toilet seats 121
Tomatoes 39, 85, 155
Tooth 171-2
   infected 172
   root canal 171
   wisdom 169
Tooth decay 171
Tooth extractions 169, 171, 173
Tooth implants 172
Townsend, John 146, 223
Trauma 1, 4, 6, 8, 134-5, 137-8, 140-2, 144, 146-7, 149, 158, 180, 223
   childhood 94, 223
Tremors 45, 61, 77, 88, 96, 153
Tricothecenes 78
TriGuard 163
Trimethylglycine 152, 175
Trust 6-7, 139, 144, 167
Tryptophan 149

TSH 15, 19
Tularemia 190, 201
Tuna 37, 149
Turkey 32, 37, 149
Twitches 45, 197

U

United Kingdom 24, 141, 216
University of Guelph 27, 216
University of Western Ontario 27
Urination, increased 77, 88
Urine 79, 93, 96, 165, 193, 209

V

Vaccinations 177
Valtrex 167
Vanilla 39
Vascular endothelial growth factor (VEGF) 88
Vasoactive Intestinal Peptide 88, 90
VCS (visual contrast sensitivity) 89-90
Vegetables 25, 32-3, 35, 38-9, 44, 128, 130, 150, 217
    cooked 12, 35-6
    green 35, 155
    juiced 35-6
    nightshade 39, 85, 155
    non-starchy 12
    starchy 38, 163
    washing 176
VEGF (vascular endothelial growth factor) 88
Venison 150
Villi 31, 34, 120, 124, 126-7, 131
VIP (vasoactive intestinal polypeptide) 88, 90
Viral encephalopathies 190
Viruses 48, 78, 113, 124, 134, 151, 159, 165, 167, 189, 200-1, 209, 211
Vitamin, corn-derived 48
Vitamin B-3 149
Vitamin B-5 50
Vitamin B-6 50, 94, 96, 99, 102, 104, 108, 148-9
Vitamin B-12 50, 152-5
Vitamin D-3 47, 176

Vitamins B-6 and B-12 175
Vomiting 100, 153, 201, 209

W

Walnuts 38, 150, 155
Watercress 39
Weakness 45, 77, 88
Weight loss 153, 207
Welchol 90
West Nile 190
Western Blot test 193
Wheat 34, 155
White blood cell 97, 99, 196, 201
White spots 95, 154
Whitehead, William 155
Wi-Fi technology 53-6, 62-3, 65, 68
Wiley, John 216
Workaholism 8
Worms 112
Wormwood 111, 119, 121, 207
Wulfman, Jeffrey 202

X

Xenoestrogens 157
Xylitol 39, 43, 91

Y

Yamuna body rolling 184, 224
Yeast overgrowth 160-3, 184
Yoga 182
Yogurt 41, 130-1
    coconut 41, 131
    goat's milk 131
    natural 32
    sheep's milk 41
Yu, Simon 111-12, 115, 119, 221

Z

Zeolite 107-8, 175-6
Zinc 49, 93-7, 99, 101-2, 104-5, 108, 148, 152, 175
Zithromax 198-9
ZYTO biocommunication machine 82, 118, 197-8